# Reflux Reality
# A Guide for Families

Written and compiled by
## Glenda Blanch
in association with the
## Reflux Infants Support Association Inc

M
A  MICHELLE ANDERSON PUBLISHING
MELBOURNE

First published in Australia 2010 by
Michelle Anderson Publishing Pty Ltd
P O Box 6032 Chapel Street North
South Yarra 3141 Melbourne
www.michelleandersonpublishing.com
mapubl@bigpond.net.au

Cover design: Chameleon Print Design
Typeset by: Midland Typesetters, Maryborough Victoria
Cover photograph: Baby Sumara and cousin Melissa
Printed by: Griffin Press, Adelaide

National Library of Australia cataloguing-in-publication entry

Author:   Blanch, Glenda,

Title:    Reflux reality: a guide for parents / Glenda Blach,
          Reflux Infants Support Association.

ISBN:     9780855723996 (pbk.)

Notes:    Bibliography.

Subjects: Gastroesophageal reflux in children.
          Gastroesophageal reflux—Treatment.

Other Authors/Contributors:
          Reflux Infants Support Association.

Dewey Number:   618.9233

# Foreword

Congratulations to Glenda Blanch and the Reflux Infants Support Association Inc for producing this fantastic book! As any mum with a newborn suffering from reflux knows, we need all the help and advice we can secure – but most of all support. This new book *Reflux Reality: A Guide for Families* has it all.

When my son Callan arrived into this world with reflux, it took me weeks to realise I was the only one in my Mums' Group who was actually getting NO sleep whatsoever. As a first-time Mum, I thought this was the normal 'sleep deprivation' aspect of babies. It did seem a little 'full on' but then everyone said babies cried a lot. Callan was vomiting after a feed (other babies seemed to do this too), but unlike some reflux babies he did not have projectile symptoms – therefore I had no idea – absolutely no idea – that anything was wrong!

As all mums of reflux babies unfortunately know, our babies don't 'sleep like a baby' and nor do their mums and dads! The impact on first-time parents, their relationship and, of course, our tiny new babies is HUGE!

I remember clearly lying on the doctor's gurney watching those fantastic scans of my son in-utero sleeping peacefully. Yet only weeks after he was born, he was the one positioned on the hospital gurney crying in pain from reflux with an ultrasound on his tiny, tiny tummy trying to work out what was wrong!

All reflux parents know our babies are very unsettled, unhappy, tired and in pain. This fantastic book containing suggested management tips, complementary medicine suggestions as well as traditional medicine, survival and coping techniques for parents and strategies to get your baby to the other side of this unwelcome health issue is hugely welcomed into the world of 21st Century Parenting.

While you are on this journey, use this wonderful book, but also remember this time does pass. Today Callan is a healthy teenager. Surprisingly I think I may even look younger than 'that' reflection in the mirror, during those long, long days and nights of getting him through reflux! He is so active, so happy, doesn't miss a trick and keeps me both on my toes AND young at heart!

Congratulations to Glenda Blanch and RISA Inc for producing this much-needed resource.

**Claudia Keech**
Founder and CEO, MotherInc
www.motherinc.com.au
Medal of the Order of Australia 2009

***

If you have tired eyes, frayed emotions, a screaming child, and thoughts of reflux then you have opened the right book! Having lived (or is that barely existed?) through reflux with both of our boys when they were babies, I know firsthand how challenging those days can be. How much more supported I would have felt if I had had a book like this to flip through! In difficult times one of the greatest gifts can be understanding. Even if you are past the worst of reflux I urge you to read this book so you can feel the acknowledgement you desperately needed. Whether you are a parent, professional or interested bystander, you will find this book easy to read, informative, and personally touching. It's the 'little golden book' for anyone involved with the impact of reflux in children.

**Felicity Chapman**
Founder and director, Mothers Be Heard
www.mothersbeheard.com

# Disclaimer

The information contained in this book is for general information and support purposes only and any similarity to your situation is purely coincidental. This information is not intended as a substitute for professional medical advice and if you have questions or concerns regarding your physical or mental health, or the health of your baby, please seek assistance from your qualified and licensed health professional. If you have any diagnosis, treatment and medication requirements, please consult a qualified and licensed health professional.

Whilst every effort is made to ensure that information contained in this book is accurate and appropriate, RISA Inc and Glenda Blanch make no warranty of any kind, express or implied, and are not liable for the accuracy, currency, errors or omissions of the information contained herein. All access to, and use of, the information is at the user's risk.

Reference herein to any specific URL or link, commercial products, process, or service by trade name, trademark, manufacturer, or otherwise is done for the convenience of the reader and does not constitute or imply its endorsement, recommendation, or favouring by RISA Inc or Glenda Blanch.

# Table of Contents

# Introduction

Chances are that if you are reading this book, your child has gastro-oesophageal reflux or you suspect they have. If you have not talked to your doctor about the possibility, it is important that you do. Even if reflux (as it is more commonly referred to) is the most likely diagnosis, it is important to rule out other conditions and confirm your suspicions before attempting strategies to help with reflux. Once the diagnosis is confirmed, you can then work with your doctor to find the most appropriate treatments for your child. This may involve trial and error because all children are different and there is no particular treatment that will work for every child.

Keep in mind that while this book aims to be a comprehensive resource, it is not a substitute for medical advice. You are encouraged to talk to your doctor or nurse whenever you have questions or concerns. You are also encouraged to trust your instincts and do what feels right, so long as it is safe. It is easy to lose confidence in yourself and your parenting abilities when your child suffers from reflux and this book may help you feel in control and better able to cope.

In the chapters ahead you will find information on reflux and management strategies, along with loads of practical advice. This includes important issues on sleeping and feeding that have been addressed in the articles and chapters written by Dr Jeanine Young, Joan Breakey and Dr Julie Cichero, all specialists in their fields. You will also find the experiences of many families as they share their insights and personal stories (identifying details have been changed in some instances). There is even a section designed specifically for family and friends to read.

Caring for a child with reflux can be time-consuming and sometimes all-encompassing, so this book is designed to be read from front to back, or section by section in any order. You can pick it up and put it down whenever you have the time – the choice is yours.

Whether your child's reflux is mild or severe, you are encouraged to choose strategies that are suitable for your situation. Remember too that medical knowledge can advance quickly, and recommended strategies can change. It is of utmost importance to keep in contact with your doctor or nurse, and keep them involved in your child's care.

## Reflux Infants Support Association (RISA) Inc

RISA Inc is a small Australian non-profit organisation that has supported reflux families since its inception in 1982. RISA Inc offers a range of services in order to provide support to families whose infants and children suffer from gastro-oesophageal reflux and its complications.

The organisation is run entirely by parents who volunteer their time to help others. Through their work it became obvious there was a real need in the community for more readily available information on reflux. This book, written by one of its members, was born in response to that need.

## About the author Glenda Blanch

I have been heavily involved in the running of this organisation for many years and have experience as a registered nurse. I am also the mother of three children who have all suffered from complications of reflux, and I suffer from reflux myself.

I was first exposed to the world of reflux twenty years ago, with the birth of our first child. Sherryn was not an easy baby; I remember feeling like a failure and wondering why everyone else coped much better than I did. I didn't know enough to put her signs together, although looking back they are obvious – the feeding and sleeping issues, (mild) irritability, recurrent throat and chest infections, wheezing and so on. Unfortunately, it was many years before she was officially diagnosed with reflux.

Our second child, Natalie, was even more difficult. Despite all the issues (and now so obvious signs), no doctor ever mentioned the possibility of reflux. She cried almost constantly, had sleeping and feeding issues, suffered frequent asthma attacks and pneumonia. She was extremely clingy, threw temper tantrums (even before she was twelve months old), and in time struggled with weight gain. The hospital became an all too familiar place, and we struggled to keep her well enough to stay home. She was four years old before she started sleeping through the night, and her reflux had still not been diagnosed!

When Anthony was born, I thought I could handle anything. I was wrong – Anthony was even more difficult. He struggled with breathing issues, rarely slept, cried lots, demanded frequent feeds, and choked and fussed throughout them (and any time in between). This at least gave us the diagnosis we desperately needed, after I woke to the sound of him choking one night. He was admitted to hospital with what doctors thought was croup, but they changed the diagnosis to gastro-oesophageal reflux disease before we went home.

At long last everything made sense, and the more I read the more sense it made. I thought that with the diagnosis, life would improve. Unfortunately, getting the diagnosis was only the first step and we tried many different treatments to find something that helped. Throughout this, life remained stressful and we often hit rock bottom. Nobody could see what was happening as Anthony was happier when we had visitors, but the constant crying, sleep deprivation, medical visits and searching for answers took over our lives. Friends as well as strangers offered endless advice, and our closest friends walked away when we were in crisis. Thankfully by then we had found RISA Inc. Having a supportive group of families to talk to, as well as accurate information about reflux and its management, made all the difference. This was even more helpful as we headed down the surgery path with Anthony and later with Natalie.

This book is not about me though. While I drew on my experiences of my reflux rollercoaster ride, and those of many other families through RISA Inc, this book is about providing you with support and information in an effort to help you on your reflux journey.

I hope it helps.

Glenda

## Reflux

The word 'reflux' is often used to describe a child's condition, whether they suffer from Gastro-Oesophageal Reflux or Gastro-Oesophageal Reflux Disease. While this can create confusion and contribute to a lack of understanding or validation within the community, many families are more comfortable with the term 'reflux' rather than the correct medical titles. For this reason, and for ease of reading, we have chosen to use the term 'reflux' predominantly throughout this book.

It is acknowledged that there is another form of reflux called Vesico-Ureteral Reflux (commonly referred to as kidney reflux); however, this book specifically focuses on Gastro-Oesophageal Reflux. Any mention of reflux is done with reference to this condition only.

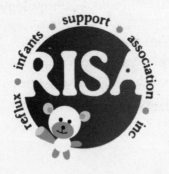

REFLUX INFANTS SUPPORT ASSOCIATION
(RISA) INC
PO Box 1598, Fortitude Valley, Qld, 4006 (Australia)
Telephone: 07 3229 1090
Website: www.reflux.org.au

# Acknowledgements

I would like to offer my sincere appreciation to everyone who contributed to this book. The number of people it has taken to put it together (even though it seemed like a simple task in the beginning) is astounding. I believe their enthusiasm and willingness to help reflects how desperately this book is needed.

I am extremely grateful to the large number of parents who contributed directly to the book or helped in any way, and particularly to Alana, Bec, Cate, Janine, Jessica, Karen and Theresa. I really appreciate their input and support.

Thanks also to everyone who has been involved in RISA Inc over the years. It is truly remarkable for parents to survive their experience, support other families AND ensure the successful running of an organisation on a totally volunteer basis. Reflux breeds remarkable people, but if you are reading this book, perhaps you already know that!

Importantly, the information compiled by many RISA Inc volunteers contributed substantially to this book – the information and their work is gratefully acknowledged.

I am also immensely grateful to all the health professionals who read and reviewed sections of the book: Professor Terry Bolin, Joan Breakey, Fiona Carter, Professor Anthony G Catto-Smith, Felicity Chapman, Dr Julie Cichero, Robyn Crapp,

Mary da Silva, Professor Elizabeth Elliott, Dr Hashem B El-Serag; Associate Professor Roger Hall OAM, Leonie Helder, Associate Professor Andrew Holland, Professor Robert Howman-Giles, Kay Hynes, Julie Maddox, Dr Sarah Manns, Dr David Manton, Heidi McLoughlin, Christine Plover, Trent Sigley, Kylie Simpson, Dr Shyan Vijayasekaran, Dr Heidi Webster and Professor (Adjunct) Jeanine Young. I also wish to thank and acknowledge the contributions provided by experts Joan Breakey, Dr Julie Cichero and Dr Jeanine Young. All the health professionals volunteered their time and expertise to ensure the information in the book is accurate, up to date, and consistent with current Australian safety guidelines. Their valued knowledge and input has added greatly to the quality of the book.

I would also like to acknowledge the help of Mr Les Priddle, Special Counsel, and thank him for his ongoing support. Thank you also to Medicare Australia and the many other organisations for their support and contribution to this book.

# Dedication

This book is dedicated to my husband Wayne and our children Sherryn, Natalie and Anthony, for their encouragement and endless patience as I worked on it. I owe them enormous thanks for allowing me to spend as much time on it as I did, for understanding its importance, and for allowing me to share our experiences. Without my wonderful family, I would never have started on my reflux journey or learnt so much, and I would not have been in a position to write this book.

With love,
Glenda

# Information on
# Gastro-oesophageal Reflux

## What is Gastro-oesophageal Reflux?

Gastro-oesophageal reflux is also known as GOR, acid reflux or gastric reflux, but it is most commonly referred to simply as reflux. It was once considered rare in children, but it is now known that reflux is a common medical issue for children of all ages. It occurs when the stomach contents (including food and stomach acid) flow into the oesophagus and sometimes out of the mouth. It is frequently seen in young infants as they regurgitate following a feed, though in some children it may also reach their lungs, sinuses or middle ear.

The stomach is able to withstand acid while the oesophagus and other areas sometimes affected by reflux (e.g. throat, nasal cavities and lungs) are generally not able to. They are easily injured if it happens often enough and this is one of the reasons why recurring reflux can cause pain, inflammation and other complications.

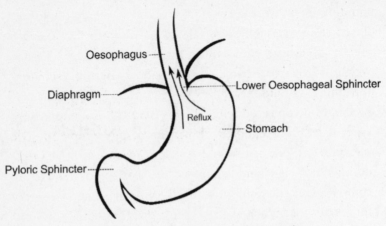

Diagram of oesophagus and stomach

## What Types of Reflux are There?

There is a lot of confusion about gastro-oesophageal reflux because the term is often used to describe the single event, the condition and the disease. The act of refluxing is the single event; it is a normal process and virtually everyone does this at times. When your child refluxes more frequently your doctor may diagnose it as gastro-oesophageal reflux, the condition. When your child has complications as a result of their reflux your doctor may diagnose it as the disease (i.e. gastro-oesophageal reflux disease).

Gastro-oesophageal reflux 'the condition' is a very common type of reflux and this is what many people think of when they picture an infant with reflux. GOR tends to peak between one and four months of age and normally resolves by two years. While it is generally more of a nuisance than a medical issue, it can still involve enormous family strains and anguish. If necessary, this form can usually be controlled by simple remedies such as thickening feeds and keeping an infant upright. It commonly presents with frequent vomiting or regurgitating but does not cause complications or long-term problems. Growth and development are normal; there is no resulting loss of weight, no extreme irritability and no significant respiratory (breathing) symptoms.

Gastro-oesophageal reflux disease (GORD) is a more severe type of reflux in children. It persists despite simple lifestyle measures and can at times be a serious medical issue. GORD occurs when signs and symptoms are severe and/or there are complications as a result of reflux; however, it is not always easy for doctors to diagnose. GORD can impact on a child's life, and they may suffer from issues such as persistent irritability, excessive vomiting or regurgitation, poor weight gain, coughing and/or feeding difficulties. GORD can be a major source of distress and concern for families and medical intervention is often necessary.

Silent reflux can add to the confusion as there may be no obvious signs of reflux. It may mean the refluxed material comes up a child's throat but is not forced out of their mouth. This has the potential to be more damaging because it can sit in the oesophagus longer than if it was vomited. Medical intervention is often necessary and the same complications can arise, but with no visible vomiting, the diagnosis can sometimes be delayed.

Laryngopharyngeal reflux (LPR) and extra-oesophageal reflux (EOR) are terms that refer to reflux that goes beyond the oesophagus. Breathing-related problems such as chronic cough, asthma, croup and/or choking can occur. The vocal cords, Eustachian tube, ears and sinuses can also be affected. A referral to a respiratory specialist or an otolaryngologist (ENT/Ear, nose and throat specialist) may be appropriate in this situation.

Whether or not there are serious medical issues to contend with as a result of your child's reflux, it can be a very stressful and overwhelming experience. If your family is in this situation, it is important you have access to the information and support you need.

## What Causes Reflux and its Complications?

Doctors do not fully understand reflux or why it causes complications in one child and not another. It is believed a combination of issues may contribute, and some are listed here:

- The lower oesophageal sphincter (a band of muscle at the lower end of the oesophagus) may not function properly. The sphincter should relax to let food and liquids into the stomach and allow burping, and then close straight away. If it stays relaxed, or relaxes at other times, stomach contents (including acid) may flow into the oesophagus. These relaxations are widely recognised as being the most common cause of reflux. Another factor for some children may be a loose or immature lower oesophageal sphincter.

- Increased pressure in the abdomen can force stomach contents into the oesophagus, especially in infants with their liquid diets. Overfeeding, straining, crying, coughing, a slumped position, or a seated position following feeds can all increase pressure in the abdomen. Tight clothes may also contribute, as can being overweight.

- Refluxed material may be cleared from the oesophagus slowly (delayed oesophageal clearance). Muscle contractions that help move food through the digestive system may be uncoordinated, weak or absent. This can expose the lining of the oesophagus to acid and other stomach contents for a longer period of time.

- The stomach may empty slowly (delayed gastric emptying), which can be a factor in reflux.
- The cells lining the oesophagus may be less resistant to damage by refluxed material. Acid combined with pepsin (a digestive enzyme made in the stomach) may cause the most damage, while bile can also damage the oesophagus.
- Genetic factors can be involved. Reflux can be an inherited condition; it is sometimes evident over different generations of the one family.
- Secondary causes of reflux can include:
  - structural issues (e.g. hiatus hernia, pyloric stenosis)
  - medical conditions that affect nerves or muscles (e.g. low muscle tone, neurological issues)
  - prematurity
  - food allergy or intolerance
  - factors that affect the lower oesophageal sphincter e.g. environmental tobacco smoke, certain medications and some foods
  - abnormal pain response in the digestive system (visceral hypersensitivity)

## What Does Reflux Look Like?

Medical advice should always be sought because reflux is not always the cause of these signs and symptoms. Healthy infants can also reflux at times.

Reflux in children shows itself in many different ways. It can range in severity from being an occasional annoyance to being severe, debilitating and sometimes even life-threatening. Reflux can improve or worsen for a variety of reasons, and your child can have good and bad days or weeks. Signs and symptoms may also depend on your child's age; this may partly relate to the fact that older children can describe their symptoms while younger children cannot (e.g. heartburn in teenagers may be the irritability and crying seen in infants).

Keep in mind that gastro-oesophageal reflux is a normal physiological event; it is termed gastro-oesophageal reflux disease when it results in harm. It can be difficult for a doctor to determine whether a child has gastro-oesophageal reflux (GOR) or gastro-oesophageal reflux disease (GORD) because signs and symptoms do not always correlate with the severity of reflux. Therefore, the following lists provide a general overview of many reflux signs, with no distinction made regarding whether they are related to GOR or GORD.

Additionally, if your child has reflux, they will not necessarily display all of the signs that are listed, and the number of signs your child has does not determine how mild or severe their reflux may be.

## Infants and Children Under the Age of Two Years

Signs and symptoms may include:
- irritability, crying, screaming
- appearing to be in pain (e.g. back-arching)
- vomiting, posseting, regurgitation
- recurrent hiccups
- wet, sour burps or hiccups
- feeding issues (e.g. refusing food or accepting only small amounts, comfort feeding)
- sleeping issues (e.g. 'catnapping', difficulty settling, night waking)
- congestion, 'snuffly' or runny nose, appearing to have a cold

- hoarse voice or different-sounding cry
- gagging, spluttering
- bad or sour-smelling breath
- weight issues (e.g. inadequate weight gain, weight loss or huge weight gains)
- frequent red throat (with infection not necessarily a factor)
- respiratory problems (e.g. choking, coughing, wheezing, chest infections)
- glue ear (fluid in the middle ear), frequent ear infections
- frequent throat or sinus infections
- drooling or excessive salivation
- gagging themselves (using their hand, fist or fingers).

## Children Between the Age of Two and Twelve Years

Children in this age group may have signs and symptoms of reflux similar to infants, or somewhere between those of infants and teenagers. They may cough, complain of pain or feeling sick, have asthma symptoms or swallowing difficulties. Your child may also not like to have any pressure on their stomach area and their behaviour may be difficult or demanding.

## Teenagers

While teenagers can display some of the previously listed signs for infants or older children, they often present similarly to adults. They may have signs and symptoms such as:

- nausea, vomiting or indigestion
- heartburn, pain or discomfort in their chest or abdomen
- feeling of a lump in their throat (or gulping after eating)
- chronic red, sore throat
- bad breath
- bitter or sour taste in their mouth

- frequent burping or throat clearing
- difficulty swallowing
- eating issues (e.g. low appetite, fussy or picky eating, constant eating or grazing)
- sleeping issues (e.g. insomnia, night-waking)
- respiratory issues (e.g. wheezing, coughing, chest infections)
- ENT issues (e.g. sinus infections, hoarseness)
- behavioural issues.

*"I learnt that children with reflux do not always complain of pain. My teenage daughter had oesophagitis despite rarely having pain, but she preferred to sleep on several pillows, woke each morning with bad breath and a cough, and wouldn't drink soft drinks (the bubbles burnt her nose when she refluxed)." Glenda*

## Common Characteristics of Reflux

In this section, parents describe some of the behaviours and characteristics that may be displayed by infants and children with reflux. Keep in mind that all children are different and the listed characteristics may not necessarily be indicative of your child's condition.

### Infants and Children Under the Age of Two Years

#### Irritability, Appearing to Be in Pain
- Irritability can cover signs such as screaming, whinging, crying and fussiness.
- Parents may have a gut feeling their child is in pain.
- Infants and children may:
  - often be distressed; however, they can still be happy

and settled at times (particularly when distracted, e.g. at the doctor or when visiting Grandma)
- arch their back, stiffen, pull their feet up or squirm
- be difficult to settle
- appear colicky or windy
- be clingy, easily upset, 'high needs' or demanding
- stick their hands, fingers or fists down their throat.

*"We were told that if Samuel was really in pain, he wouldn't stop crying if I picked him up, and often he didn't, but other times he did, especially if I held him upright. I think they associate their Mums with comfort, so they feel better just by being picked up." Karen*

*"It's so frustrating when our children smile at everyone even if they have spent the entire day crying. Nobody sees how bad things really are!" Glenda*

## Vomiting, Posseting or Regurgitation

- Infants and children who vomit can:
  - regurgitate or posset (down their chin and or clothing)
  - projectile vomit with food literally being forced out, sometimes through their nostrils.
- Vomit can appear to contain:
  - milk, food or other stomach contents (e.g. stomach acid, mucous)
  - blood (may look like coffee grounds, or be black or red, with streaks or clots)
  - bile (can appear green or yellow).
- The number and amount of vomits can vary, but it often occurs after feeds.

- They may vomit without discretion anytime, anywhere, over anybody or anything.

**Feeding Issues**
- Infants and children with feeding difficulties may:
  - pull away from the breast/bottle after a short time, push the breast/bottle away, stiffen up, squirm or arch their back
  - scream and refuse to feed (or take only small amounts despite being hungry)
  - become easily distracted, nervous or excitable; even people talking may interrupt their feed
  - display a fear of food, an unwillingness to eat or be particularly fussy
  - feed only when drowsy or asleep
  - gag/splutter or have problems swallowing
  - have difficulties with some textures
  - be happy between feeds
  - have allergies or intolerances to particular foods.
- Infants and children who 'comfort feed' may:
  - feed frequently or be unhappy unless feeding
  - suck vigorously
  - have huge weight gains
  - have a large number of wet nappies due to their frequent feeding.

*"In the beginning, Ewan was a 'happy chucker'. Whilst he was a miserable baby he did not scream or cry when projectile vomiting. I was lulled into the false sense that he was okay because everyone focused on the vomiting and not the feeding*

*problems, back arching, leg pulling up, etc. I wish I had been alerted to these being signs of severe reflux." Janine*

## Sleeping Issues
- Infants and children may:
  - be more comfortable in a fully upright position and may object to lying down, particularly after a feed
  - take short naps (catnaps) and may wake distressed
  - be restless or easily disturbed from sleep
  - have trouble self-settling
  - wake frequently overnight (although some infants with reflux sleep through the night – they may simply be exhausted or may not reflux much overnight).

## Weight Issues
- Weight issues may not necessarily reflect the severity of a child's reflux. Infants and children can have significant reflux, even with normal weight and weight gains.
- Most infants with reflux gain weight well; however, some infants do not gain weight at the expected rate and may fail to thrive. This may be a result of feeding difficulties, frequent vomiting or other issues.
- Some reflux infants have large weight gains, particularly if they feed frequently.

## Other Characteristics
- Reflux can be cyclic. Infants and children can go through normal phases where issues appear to be improving and then recur suddenly, sometimes for no apparent reason.
- Parents often report a worsening of their child's reflux with illnesses, teething, crawling, vaccinations, constipation, being overtired or out of routine. They also report that hot

humid weather can be a trigger, as can laughing, jumping, running, playing games and other physical activities.

*"Jorja went back on medications for reflux when she got her first tooth last month – the combination of teeth, crawling, hot weather and a virus all took their toll. She didn't vomit like before – just endless crying, burps, neck arching, not sleeping."* Trudi

- Signs of reflux may change as infants and children get older. It can look as though their reflux is improving because their signs go away, but their signs may have changed instead (e.g. your child may no longer vomit but they can still be refluxing significantly).
- Infants and children may:
  - gag, splutter or swallow even when not feeding
  - stop babbling or talking, perhaps in response to pain
  - not be easily distracted and may need lots of physical contact
  - develop behavioural issues
  - have teeth that show signs of erosion.
- Responses may be unpredictable; what works one day may not work the next.

## Children Over the Age of Two Years and Teenagers

Most children seem to grow out of reflux before the age of two years, but some continue to suffer from reflux beyond that. While the previously listed characteristics may still be relevant, they may also display some of the following characteristics.

- Even if a child seems to have outgrown reflux, parents sometimes report it recurs at times of stress (e.g. exams, starting school) or when reflux often flares e.g. teething.

- Children may verbalise how they feel (e.g. "My tummy/throat hurts", "I feel sick").
- Children may display behavioural issues and may:
  - cry easily or 'lose the plot' over small issues
  - be easily irritated or moody
  - have temper tantrums (either extreme or outside the normal age range)
  - be aggressive or display violent behaviour
  - have severe separation anxiety
  - be impossible or difficult to reason with
  - be unpredictable (e.g. will play happily in a group one day and be withdrawn the next)
  - harm themselves (e.g. head-banging, obsessive nail-biting.

*"Anything can send him to tears; if another child TALKS to him he can start to cry." Jules*

*"Anthony was aggressive because of his reflux. When his reflux was finally controlled, he was the most gorgeous, placid child; the change in him was amazing." Glenda*

- Children may have eating issues and may:
  - have food aversions, or sensitivities to different textures
  - demand water frequently; some drink fluids in preference to eating
  - refuse to eat; some refuse breakfast but eat lunch (though some are the opposite and refuse meals later in the day)
  - prefer to snack constantly rather than eat regular meals.

- Children may have sleeping issues and:
  - have difficulty falling asleep
  - want lots of pillows to sleep on (they may not like to lie flat)
  - be restless during sleep, or may cry, moan or swallow even while asleep
  - ask (or be desperate) for drinks of water overnight or immediately on waking.
- Children may:
  - appear to be in pain (e.g. they may hold their tummy or double over)
  - appear tired or lethargic
  - have a hoarse or croaky voice, especially on waking
  - burp frequently
  - look pale
  - have motion sickness
  - have difficulty concentrating or paying attention
  - not necessarily be aware of their reflux, especially if it has been an ongoing issue.
- Therapies used to correct any issues (e.g. behaviour, eating or sleeping) may be ineffective until the underlying cause is addressed.

*"Children with reflux can present differently, even in the same family." Sharon*

## Complications of Reflux

If reflux episodes are excessive, severe or persistent, your child may experience complications (i.e. gastro-oesophageal reflux disease). When this occurs, a vicious cycle can follow, causing more reflux. Some complications are listed here:

- Oesophagitis (a red, irritated and/or ulcerated oesophagus) occurs when acidic stomach contents burn or irritate the lining of the oesophagus. This can cause pain, nausea or blood in vomit and/or faeces (your child's 'poo'); however, there may be no obvious signs or symptoms.
  - Longstanding reflux with inflammation or irritation can cause scarring, thickening or narrowing of the oesophagus (stricture) and swallowing difficulties.
  - If the damage goes unchecked in longstanding reflux, it may develop into a rare condition called Barrett's Oesophagus. The body tries to protect itself from the chronic reflux and changes cells in the lining of the lower oesophagus. These new cells are abnormal, though the reason for this is not yet understood.
- Oral aversion: Infants and children may learn to associate eating or drinking with pain, discomfort or nausea and so may choose not to eat. It may be the food itself or the reflux that occurs with a feed that causes the distress, and therapy may be needed to address the issue. Some children also become overly sensitive or agitated in response to different touch or textures anywhere near their mouth or face.
- Failure to thrive (FTT) or poor growth may be the result of significant vomiting and/or refusal to eat. Alternatively, food sensitivities can impair the body's ability to absorb nutrients, and the loss of a specific food group without a dietitian's guidance can lead to failure to thrive. Severe failure to thrive can necessitate the child being fed by tube.
- Respiratory (breathing) issues may be associated with

aspiration (breathing in food or reflux matter into the lungs) or stimulation of the nerves causing issues such as wheezing, stridor (harsh breathing sound), coughing, croup, frequent chest infections, and sometimes apnoea (a pause in breathing) or cyanosis (turning blue or grey). *Please note: if your child has any breathing difficulties, seek urgent medical advice.*

- Recurrent ear, throat and/or sinus infections or other related issues can be a complication of reflux.
- Iron-deficiency anaemia can result from feeding issues, poor iron absorption, oesophagitis or chronic bleeding in the oesophagus.
- Dental erosion may be a factor because teeth may be repeatedly exposed to stomach acid.
- Developmental delays may be an issue because of pain, lack of sleep, excessive crying or a lack of tummy time.
- Sandifer's syndrome or torticollis: Abnormal head and neck posturing or neck tilting is thought to be a response to pain, or the body's way of protecting the airway from reflux material. It can sometimes be mistaken for seizures if repetitive movements are made.

*"Bella displayed Sandifer's syndrome posturing . . . until she was medicated. Sometimes if I was holding her facing my chest, she'd try to almost bend over backwards in half." Jess*

## Growing Out of Reflux

There are many different theories about when children grow out of reflux and you may be told specific times (e.g. three or six months). Unfortunately, the reality is that it is not possible to predict. Most infants seem to improve significantly throughout their first twelve months as they become increasingly upright, develop strength in their abdomen and later as their slowing growth rate results in the need for less food. However, reflux may continue to be an issue for some children (even if they seem to have outgrown it), and further studies are needed in this area.

Certain milestones may bring considerable improvement and there is always hope that your child will improve earlier rather than later. In the meantime, it may help to focus on managing your child's reflux and taking each day as it comes.

## Common Myths About Reflux in Children

There are a lot of myths surrounding gastro-oesophageal reflux in children and some common ones are listed below. Please be guided by your instincts and talk to your doctor or nurse if you have any concerns.

### 1. Myth: Reflux is just another name for colic.
**Reality:** Colic is not a well-understood condition and medical research into it is continuing. It is known, though, that there may be many possible causes for it and that some infants who display colicky behaviour may have reflux and/or a milk protein allergy. It is also possible that some cases of colic may be undiagnosed reflux.

### 2. Myth: All babies have reflux; it's no big deal.
**Reality:** It is true that almost all babies reflux occasionally without causing harm, as many people are aware. However, there is a huge difference between occasional episodes of reflux and reflux that causes complications (GORD). For children who have GORD (and their families), it can be a very big deal. Unfortunately, many people know this condition as 'reflux' and do not realise it can sometimes be a very serious issue.

**3. Myth: If you are having problems, it is because you are inexperienced or doing something wrong. "Is this your first child?"**

**Reality:** Issues with sleeping, feeding, development and behaviour are common in children with reflux, and caring for them can be extremely stressful and overwhelming even for experienced parents. It does not mean you are doing anything wrong if your child has problems; it may just mean you have not yet found the answers you need.

**4. Myth: Children have to look sick or cry all the time to have reflux. "She always looks happy to me"; "But he looks so healthy!"**

**Reality:** Some children with reflux appear to be quite happy at times, especially if they are distracted (e.g. by an outing, with visitors or at the doctor's). This can make it difficult for families to get the treatment or understanding that is needed. A child with reflux who looks happy and healthy to others generally looks that way because their families spend most of their time trying to make sure they are!

**5. Myth: If an infant gains weight well, their reflux is not serious or worth treating.**

**Reality:** Some infants with reflux have issues with their growth and may even have failure to thrive. However, others have no growth concerns and some have huge weight gains. These infants can still suffer from severe reflux and other complications, but because their growth is not a concern their condition may not be taken seriously and the treatment they need may sometimes be delayed.

# 2

# Medical Information

## Medical Advice

It is important to discuss any concerns with your medical health professional. A variety of conditions can cause vomiting and other reflux-like symptoms in infants and children (such as urinary tract infection, pyloric stenosis, coeliac disease) and your child should only be regarded as having gastro-oesophageal reflux or gastro-oesophageal reflux disease when their doctor makes that diagnosis. Additionally, the majority of newborn babies vomit at some stage and in most cases no further investigation or treatment is necessary.

The first step in treating your child is to seek medical advice, even if reflux seems like an obvious diagnosis or your child is otherwise healthy and happy. This is important as early diagnosis and appropriate treatment may improve a child's quality of life and long-term health.

If your doctor diagnoses reflux, it is important you are provided with information about the condition and what to expect, as well as the initial plan for management and investigations (if indicated). Reassurance can be enormously helpful and in some circumstances may be all that you need; however, there may also be a lot of issues you would like to discuss with your doctor.

## Discussing Issues with Your Doctor

It is easy to lose confidence in yourself and your parenting ability when you have a child with reflux. As a result, you may find discussing concerns with your doctor very daunting.

Keep in mind you are not wasting your doctor's time if you have concerns about your child. It is not your role as a parent to know the answers; your role is to bring concerns to your doctor's attention. If nothing else, this can give you peace of mind.

Your doctor will be able to listen to what you say, ask pertinent questions and perhaps diagnose reflux (if that has not already been done). However, it may not be this simple, especially if your child does not vomit/regurgitate. Your child's signs and symptoms may fit with other conditions, or your doctor may consider them to be within normal range. If this is the case and your instincts tell you something is wrong, it is important you pursue it.

There are strategies you can use so you feel confident your doctor understands the situation. Being prepared for the appointment can help, and some of the following suggestions may be useful. Try to remain calm if possible, as this may help you communicate more clearly with your doctor (but also let your doctor know if you are feeling depressed or unable to cope). Finally, do not be discouraged if your child is crying or unsettled at the appointment as this may be a good opportunity for your doctor to see what is happening firsthand.

- Have clear goals. Think about what you want from your doctor before the appointment.
- Make a list of all your concerns so you can present them in a clear, organised way. Consider areas your doctor may ask about (e.g. sleeping, feeding, behaviour), and think about how you will respond. Your child's reflux signs may not be apparent during the short appointment time and it is important your doctor understands the entire issue.
  - Writing a list of your child's signs and symptoms, including when they occur and how long they last, may help. You may wish to use information from the previous chapter as a guide.
- Have a checklist of what you want to discuss, including your child's medical history, treatments you have tried and any other points that seem relevant.
- Keep a written diary for at least twenty-four hours before the appointment (longer if possible). Record details of feeds and sleep patterns, times your child is unsettled or distressed, vomiting or other reflux behaviours, and any other issues. If you are breastfeeding, include what you eat and drink as well.
- Bring your partner, family member or friend with you to the appointment. They can confirm any issues, take note of what your doctor says and attend to your child if necessary. A letter from someone who has witnessed any issues may also help (e.g. carer at your child's daycare centre).
- Book a long appointment if you have a lot to discuss, so your doctor can give adequate attention to the issues. Be aware that further appointments may be necessary.
- Be as truthful as you can. If your doctor does not seem to understand your concerns, do not be tempted to exagger-

ate or stretch the truth as this can undermine anything you say.

- Take video footage of your child's symptoms or behaviours, and show your doctor.

*"James is worse at night (less distractions) and after his last breastfeed . . . [I] have decided to pull out the video camera, film a night-time feeding session and send it to my paediatrician." Jessica*

- Ask for further details if you have questions or are unsure of anything.
- Ask for information or instructions to be written down for you, or take notes. It can sometimes be difficult to recall specific details.
- Ask your doctor if they have any printed material available, and ask where you can go for further support or information.

Also, find out how to best contact your doctor if your child worsens in the days following the appointment, especially if you are trying something new. It may also help if you organise another appointment so you can discuss further issues or concerns.

If you feel your doctor does not understand what you are trying to convey, seem to have enough experience or offer the information and support you need, you have the option of pursuing it with them or seeking another opinion. Keep in mind that no doctor knows everything about every subject. Depending on the situation, a referral to a paediatrician, paediatric gastroenterologist or other specialist may be necessary.

*"I believe a mother should always follow her instincts (ninety-nine percent of the time she's right) so if you think your baby has a problem, be persistent and push for answers."* Alana

*"You are your child's advocate. Don't be afraid to ask questions and push for answers if you need to."*

*"Some specialists have long waiting lists but you can ask if they have a cancellation list. Your referring doctor can also ask for an earlier appointment if it's urgent."*

## Reflux Is Not Always To Blame

Be aware that reflux is not always to blame for every issue. If your child is distressed or unwell, it is important not to jump to conclusions. Even if your child does suffer from reflux, it may not always be the culprit.

*"[My son] was so unsettled and wouldn't eat and was vomiting more. I was sure it was his reflux but I thought I'd take him to the GP . . . it turned out both his ears were quite bad[ly infected]."*

## When to Especially Seek Medical Advice

Always seek medical advice if you have any concerns about your child or yourself. In relation to reflux, you should seek medical advice especially if there are any issues such as:
- Your infant or child:
  - is very irritable, cries excessively or is inconsolable
  - appears to be in pain
  - has sleeping issues
  - has weight loss or poor weight gain
  - appears to be refluxing frequently.
- Your child complains of:

- food/fluid coming up into their throat or mouth
- heartburn or pain in the stomach or chest area
- difficult or painful swallowing
- food getting stuck.
- Your infant or child's vomiting or regurgitation:
  - is of large volume or frequent
  - is increasing in amount
  - is forceful
  - contains coffee ground-like material or is black, red or brown
  - is green or yellow.
- With feeding, your infant or child:
  - refuses to eat/feed
  - pulls off the breast or bottle, or frequently interrupts the feed
  - is difficult to reattach to the breast or bottle
  - arches their back, draws their legs up or screams
  - is fussy or sensitive to different textures
  - chokes or gags
  - complains of pain.
  
  *(See the chapter on 'Feeding: A Speech Pathologist's Perspective' for further information)*
- Your infant or child has chest problems:
  - any increased breathing effort or difficulty breathing, particularly after vomiting or during/after eating
  - repeated coughing
  - wheezing
  - repeated chest infections or pneumonia
  - apnoeas (breathing stops temporarily)
  - cyanosis (turning blue) or colour changes (turning pale or blue) around their mouth or face.

- You and/or your partner are:
  - distressed
  - overtired and exhausted
  - confused about how to manage your child
  - lacking support
  - socially isolated because of your child's behaviour
  - depressed or feeling down/negative
  - not eating
  - not sleeping
  - not coping
  - excessively weepy
  - worried that you might harm your child or yourself.

## Hospitalisation

Children with reflux can be hospitalised for a variety of reasons. These may include:

- observation
- commencement or alteration of treatment
- establishing a feeding pattern
- investigations or procedures (e.g. endoscopy, surgery)
- for treatment of reflux complications (e.g. asthma, chest infections, refusal to feed)
- to give the family temporary respite from the distress they are experiencing.

## Medical Investigations and Procedures

While investigations are not always required for the diagnosis of reflux, they can be useful in some circumstances (e.g. to document the occurrence of reflux, or evaluate the effectiveness of treatment). Each test is designed to answer a specific question and is valuable only when used in the appropriate situation. They may not necessarily exclude reflux or its complications, even if the results are negative.

If your child is undergoing any investigation, it may help if you know why your doctor wants it performed, what they want to learn from it and whether it is likely to change your child's treatment. It may also help if you know what to expect on the day, how long the test will take and whether you can be present, so if you have any questions, do not hesitate to ask.

You will be provided with specific information and instructions for the procedure at the time of booking (e.g. whether your child should have nothing to eat or drink beforehand, and if medication should be stopped). Instructions may depend on factors such as the hospital/x-ray department's protocol, your child's age and capabilities, whether they are breastfed, and the aim of the investigation.

If your child is old enough, you may need to consider what to tell them. It may be enough to give basic explanations but older children may appreciate more information. Talk to your doctor if you are unsure what to say.

It may help your child if you bring a special toy or activity with you. They may also feel more comfortable if you stay with them (if possible), and on the day of the test you may prefer to have a support person with you too.

## Fasting for Investigations

Many investigations or procedures require your child to have no food or milk for several hours beforehand (often referred to as 'fasting'). This safety precaution is done to protect your child's lungs by minimising their risk of aspirating or regurgitating stomach contents into their lungs during the procedure. You will be advised if fasting is necessary for each test and if so, for how long. Fasting times are generally shorter if your child is breastfed, as breastmilk empties from the stomach much faster than infant formula.

## Barium Swallow

A barium swallow is a series of x-rays taken as your child swallows barium (a white, chalky liquid that shows up on x-ray). It coats your child's oesophagus, stomach and small intestine. This allows the doctor to see the outline of these organs and, importantly, whether your child's anatomy is normal. It can also reveal other conditions such as a hiatus hernia.

A barium swallow is a short test. Even if your child has significant gastro-oesophageal reflux, they may not reflux during the procedure and so a 'normal' result may not necessarily exclude reflux or its complications. Additionally, an episode of reflux captured during testing may simply be a single reflux episode and is not diagnostic of gastro-oesophageal reflux disease.

The test is performed with your child lying on a table underneath an x-ray machine. This machine is linked to a nearby screen so that the x-ray image can be seen as the barium is swallowed. Very young children may be given the barium mixture through a bottle or syringe, while older children may be offered it in a cup with flavouring of some sort. In some circumstances, a nasogastric tube may be inserted so they receive the barium.

Your child may be placed (or asked to move) in different positions so the barium coats their organs well. X-rays are taken as the barium passes through your child's upper digestive tract. Once this is done, the test is complete and your child can return to normal daily activities. Fluids are encouraged to help the barium pass through their system as it can cause constipation.

*"Anthony had a barium swallow when he was eleven weeks old. I found it all pretty difficult, especially as he was so young, but*

*thankfully the test itself didn't take too long. He had to go without a feed for several hours before the test, which wasn't easy as he was a comfort feeder and demanded feeds quite frequently. He was laid down on the x-ray table, and given a bottle with barium in it. He'd never had a bottle, but he managed to get enough in to do the test. They took a few x-rays as he drank, and watched the barium on a nearby screen. They picked up that he was refluxing, but saw no other abnormalities." Glenda*

## Modified Barium Swallow

A modified barium swallow, as its name suggests, is performed in a similar manner to a barium swallow; however, it is performed by a speech pathologist and radiologist. Its major aim is to look in detail at the mouth (oral stage), throat (pharyngeal stage) and then sometimes down towards the oesophagus, which are areas that are sometimes missed in a barium swallow. It is used to determine if your child swallows safely and also what types of food or fluids are safe for them. Your child will be given food or fluids with barium to swallow and their ability to swallow will be assessed. The speech pathologist then provides recommendations for safe food textures and fluid thickness levels and may also provide advice on swallowing strategies.

## Upper Endoscopy

An upper endoscopy is an examination of the lining of the oesophagus, stomach, and upper duodenum with a flexible fibre-optic tube (endoscope). The doctor is able to view the lining of these organs and take photos and/or biopsies (tissue samples) for review under the microscope. This test is helpful in determining the condition of the upper digestive tract, if there is any inflammation or ulcers in the oesophagus and sometimes how well the lower oesophageal sphincter works.

It is performed under general anaesthetic so your child will need to be admitted to hospital for this procedure. Once your child is asleep, the doctor very carefully inserts the endoscope through your child's mouth and into their oesophagus. An image can be seen on a nearby screen, and photographs or biopsies are sometimes taken. Following the procedure, which generally takes from fifteen to thirty minutes, your child will be under observation in a recovery room or ward for several hours. You may be encouraged to be with your child as they wake.

*"We arrived in the morning, got checked in, saw the nurse and anaesthetist, then went into the procedure (they do them from youngest to oldest). I got to stay with my daughter while they put the mask on for the anaesthetic, then I went out and it only took twenty minutes and they were finished." Mary*

## pH Probe

A pH probe demonstrates episodes of acid reflux including how often they occur, how long they last, and whether they are related to signs like coughing, irritability and vomiting. It can be useful to show the presence of acid reflux if it is not demonstrated by other investigations, and also determine the effectiveness of treatment. A pH probe may not be indicated if reflux is obvious, and a negative result does not necessarily exclude the condition or its symptoms.

A thin, flexible tube with a pH sensor is passed through your child's nose and positioned in their oesophagus. An x-ray is taken to ensure the tube is correctly placed. It is then taped securely to your child's cheek and attached to a portable record-ing device.

It can be very uncomfortable for your child as the tube is being passed. However, once it is in position the tube is usually well tolerated and your child should be able to eat and sleep quite normally. Some children, especially if they are young, will need splints on their arms to prevent them from pulling the tubing out. They may be able to go home with the tube in place, or they may be admitted to hospital, depending on hos-pital policy and the situation.

The tube is generally left in place for twenty-four hours and the recorded data is then downloaded and analysed. Any acid reflux (pH less than four) that occurs is expressed as a percent-age of the total recording time.

> *"Anthony was three years old when he had a pH probe. He gagged while the tubing was being inserted but settled pretty quickly. It was x-rayed and then taped in place. The monitor was placed in our backpack and we went home. I recorded when he ate, drank, lay down or seemed to reflux (e.g. cough, com-plain of pain). We returned to the hospital the next day to have it removed and we received the results several days later."* Glenda

## Multichannel Intraluminal Impedance (MII)/pH Monitoring

Impedance monitoring, combined with pH monitoring, records both acid and non-acid reflux. This significantly improves the correlation of symptoms with reflux episodes including how often they occur, how long they last, and also whether they are related to signs like coughing, irritability and vomiting. This technology can be especially useful when evaluating children with less typical symptoms (e.g. breathing issues).

Combined oesophageal pH/impedance monitoring is performed in a similar manner to a pH probe. A tube is inserted through the child's nose and connected to a small computer. This tube has sensors that measure changes in pressure (impedance) and others that measure pH. After twenty-four hours, the recording is downloaded and analysed.

## Oesophageal Manometry

Oesophageal manometry is a test that helps to identify if there are any issues getting food or fluid into your child's stomach after it is swallowed. It provides information about the tone (pressure) and peristalsis (wave patterns) in the oesophagus and the tone of the lower oesophageal sphincter.

A thin pressure-sensitive tube is passed through your child's nose and into their oesophagus (in a similar manner to a pH probe), and then attached to a computer and specialised equipment. The wave patterns and pressures are recorded during rest periods and when your child swallows food or water. The test takes approximately two hours to complete.

## Milk Scan

A milk scan studies the period of time immediately following a meal, and involves adding tiny amounts of radioactive materials (radioisotopes) into your child's body via their milk. A computer and special camera are used to take pictures and track the milk as it is swallowed. It is useful in demonstrating both acid and non-acid reflux, and may also help determine whether aspiration (spill over into the lungs) is present and how long milk or food sits in your child's stomach (gastric emptying study).

The technologist will add radioisotopes to your child's milk, breastmilk or formula (the radioisotopes do not change its taste or smell). It will then be given to your child to drink. In some circumstances (e.g. if your child has swallowing difficulties) a nasogastric tube may be inserted so the milk can be given.

Your child will then lie on a table in the examination room, while the camera takes a series of pictures to track the movement of the radioisotopes. This will continue for approximately an hour, and once this is done the test is complete. Your child may wish to watch a DVD or video while the test is being performed, and they may feel more comfortable if you stay in the examination room with them. Once the pictures are taken, your child will be able to return to their usual activities.

## Tracheal Pepsin Assay

Tracheal pepsin assay is a procedure that is used to determine if aspiration into the lungs is occurring. A sample of secretions is taken from your child's windpipe (trachea) when they are under general anaesthetic, and then tested for pepsin (an enzyme made in the stomach). Its presence in the windpipe is thought to confirm reflux in the lungs.

# 3

# An Overview of
# Managing Reflux

## Treating Reflux

Gastro-oesophageal reflux requires a thorough medical assessment before a diagnosis can be made. Once reflux is diagnosed, the type of treatment needed will be determined, taking into account the severity of your child's reflux, any complications, and the age of your child. From a medical point of view, because there is no cure for reflux, treatments are generally aimed at improving symptoms, healing any inflammation and preventing complications.

All children with reflux are different. Medical advice and reassurance is sometimes all that is necessary, but for others, finding the right treatment can take time. For many, the first line of treatment includes lifestyle changes (also called conservative treatments). Strategies such as avoiding overfeeding, changing diet, avoiding the seated position immediately after feeding and eliminating exposure to tobacco smoke have been shown to improve symptoms in many infants with reflux.

If your child's symptoms are severe or persistent, your doctor may consider treatment with medication or referral to a paediatrician or paediatric gastroenterologist for further evaluation. Also, doctors may occasionally use medication for a limited period of time to help determine if a child's symptoms are due to reflux. Surgery may be an option for a very small number of children with reflux.

Nurses, allied health professionals (e.g. speech therapists, dietitians) and complementary medicine therapists (e.g. naturopaths) may also play a role, depending on the issues being faced and family circumstances. Treating constipation at any age can also be helpful in reducing reflux episodes.

*"I learnt from experience to try one thing at a time, as otherwise you don't know what is working." Kylie*

## Summary of Lifestyle Changes

The following strategies are often recommended in the treatment of reflux in infants and children. Lifestyle changes may help to control your child's reflux or make them feel more comfortable, and even if medications are used, these strategies may still be helpful. See the following chapters for more detailed information.

### Infants and Children Under the Age of Two Years

- Seek medical advice about any concerns. It is important you are listened to and believed, and provided with the reassurance and information you need.
- Avoid secondhand smoke. Tobacco smoke can relax the lower oesophageal sphincter and make reflux more likely. It can also make infants more irritable and cause irritation to the oesophagus and lungs.

- Feed your infant in an upright position if possible, and try to keep them upright for at least thirty minutes after each feed. Try to avoid the upright seated position during this time as this position can increase pressure in the abdomen.
- Avoid placing your infant flat on their back immediately following a feed.
- Try feeding smaller amounts more often, unless this upsets your infant. Large feeds given frequently can cause reflux.
- Burp a breastfed infant after they finish feeding on each side, and burp a bottle-fed infant after every thirty to sixty millilitres they drink (as tolerated).
- Avoid overfeeding. It is not recommended to feed infants again if they vomit, but to wait until the next feed. Talk to your doctor or child-health nurse to ensure your infant is taking appropriate amounts of food.
- Thickened feeds may be effective for some infants, especially those who vomit.
- If a food allergy or intolerance is suspected, a two-week trial of hypoallergenic formula can be helpful if your infant is formula-fed. If you are breastfeeding you may, with medical supervision, choose to eliminate specific foods (e.g. cow's milk and soy) from your diet.
- Minimise foods and drinks if they cause irritation or increase the risk of reflux. Examples of these may be spicy foods, citrus fruits, tomatoes and other acidic food, fatty foods and caffeine.
- Avoid tight nappies and elastic waistbands, and ensure clothing around abdominal area is loose fitting.
- If you are comfortable considering this, offer your infant a dummy/pacifier (or your clean finger), as non-nutritive sucking may help your infant to settle.

- If your child is over the age of twelve months, sleeping them on their left side may reduce reflux. From birth to twelve months, the side-sleeping position is *not* stable, increases the risk of sudden unexpected death in infancy, and is not recommended.
- If your child is under the age of twelve months, elevating the head of the bed to treat reflux is not supported by evidence from research studies. It may reduce reflux in some children who are over twelve months of age.

## Children Over the Age of Two Years and Teenagers

Many of the lifestyle changes can be adapted for older children. Depending on the child and their age, they should be offered an explanation and reassurance. They could also be helped and encouraged to:

- Have good eating habits and make healthy decisions. It will help to have healthy food prepared, and also for your child to see the rest of the family participating. Older children may like to participate in the shopping, meal preparation and cooking.
- Eat smaller meals more frequently.
- Avoid lying down or going to bed for several hours after eating.
- Avoid big meals, especially before exercising, bedtime or stressful events such as exams.
- Consider the possibility of food allergy or intolerance, in particular to cow's milk protein. Seek medical advice regarding this.
- Minimise foods and drinks (including alcohol) if they cause irritation or increase the risk of reflux.
- Avoid exposure to cigarette/tobacco smoke.

- Avoid or minimise caffeine. Caffeine can be found in tea, coffee, energy drinks, some soft drinks (e.g. colas), cocoa and some over-the-counter medications.
- Wear comfortable, loose clothing.
- Lose weight if overweight, or seek medical advice regarding weight loss.
- Sleep with the head of the bed elevated as it may reduce reflux episodes in this age group.
- Find a comfortable sleeping position. Sleeping in the prone position (on the tummy) may be helpful for children in this age group as it may reduce episodes of reflux. Sleeping on the left side may also be helpful in older children.
- Consider using sugar-free chewing gum after meals; it may reduce acid reflux and help clear acid from the oesophagus.
- Avoid medications that can be irritating to the gut. This should be discussed with the doctor.

## General Home Management Tips

### Tips for Managing Vomiting

Further treatment beyond lifestyle changes may not be necessary if your infant or child regurgitates or vomits a lot, providing they are happy, feeding well, putting on appropriate amounts of weight and reaching their milestones appropriately. However, this can be frustrating and difficult for you to accept (if your child does vomit) and the vomiting itself can become stressful and overwhelming. There may be an enormous amount of extra washing, which may include your child's clothes, bedding, your own clothing, and even furniture. The embarrassment from all the vomiting and the expense from extra washing can also be difficult to manage. Furthermore, you may avoid going out, or may restrict your social activities because of your child's vomiting.

*"My biggest issue with reflux: VOMITING! Both boys were huge vomiters and would often be vomiting when I had to put them to bed. They would only ever sleep for forty minutes then wake up in a pool of vomit." Nelle*

You may find the suggestions below helpful; however, if you are concerned about any vomiting, or your child is struggling to put on weight or reach their milestones, it is important you seek medical advice.

- Have lots of bibs handy. Use large bibs rather than those young infant ones designed to catch small dribbles.
- A square of material with plastic/waterproof backing is a good puddle mat to lay your infant on at home or when visiting. Place it on your lap whilst feeding as personal protection, or use towels.

*"I would take plastic-backed picnic blankets with us when we went to visit anyone, to use on the floor."*

- A cloth or sheet over the feeding chair can save extra cleaning of upholstery and carpets. Alternatively, reduce stress and feed on an old lounge or wooden (easily cleaned) chair.

*"I kept a pile of cloth nappies on the armrest of the chair I was feeding on. I then covered the lounge and myself with cloth nappies to mop up spills." Nelle*

- Lay towels or a large wipe-clean mat on the floor next to the cot to protect the flooring. It may also help to lay a plastic sheet underneath the towels.

- Have lots of cloths (e.g. a large pack or two of cloth nappies) or a supply of towels handy, to wipe up spills. Cover the lounge with them and put them under your infant's head when they are nursing or burping.

*"I used cloth nappies . . . [they are] nice and soft against their face and can also wipe the remaining mess. Easy to wash and reuse." Trudi*

- Make your child's bed with several layers of sheets, separated by waterproof sheets. It is quicker and easier to take the top layer off when they need to be changed. Ensure safe sleeping guidelines for safe infant bedding are followed, available at www.sidsandkids.org.
- Feed on an easily cleanable floor, plastic sheet or outside on the grass to minimise work. Try feeding in the bath for a change.

*"We are renting and the endless mess on the carpet stressed me, so we bought some cheap rugs to cover the carpet . . . Sure we still cleaned up vomit, but we didn't worry as much." Anna*

- Have lots of changes of clothes available for your infant, but even so, try to change them only when necessary. This may minimise your infant's distress and help reduce the amount they vomit.
- Wear old clothes so you do not get too upset when vomit and/or medications get on them.

*"Vomit stains are hidden better on patterned clothing but seem to stand out a lot on plain T-shirts."*

- Protect your child's skin from all the vomiting or drooling by using a protective cream.

- Using a stain-inhibitor product on your furniture and quick cleaning may prevent staining.
- Have a bucket of nappy soaker in the laundry sink to toss smelly clothes and wipe-up cloths in so they do not stain.
- Try to ensure your child's environment is easy to clean, and toys and equipment are easy to wipe over or wash (e.g. highchair tray is easy to remove).
- A paste of bicarbonate of soda and water spread on fabric may help remove the odour of vomit. Fabric refresher spray may help on fabric that is not washable. Keep a spray bottle with water and bicarbonate of soda handy to absorb smells.
- To remove the odour of vomit (and other nasty smells) that can linger on hands even after thorough washing, try smearing toothpaste on them and then rinsing off.

*"The quick-dry gym or hair towels are great for carrying around when travelling as they don't take up as much room in your bag as cloth nappies." Nelle*

## Having a Successful Outing with Your Child

Outings can be difficult if you have a child with reflux. Some tips you may find helpful are listed below:

- Where possible arrange outdoor outings, reducing the likelihood of having to wipe up any vomit and the embarrassment that goes with it. The fresh air can work wonders.

*"I don't like leaving the house on my own. Who would, with a screaming baby? . . . But I must say I do feel better when I get out. Even for a walk." Sharon*

- Take changes of clothes for you and your child, as well as laundry bags.

*"Always carry a towel, bucket and a change of clothing in the boot of the car . . . [we] use it at LEAST once a week." Shell*

- Being carried in a baby sling/backpack keeps them upright and can offer your child lots of stimuli. Use it for any outings (e.g. grocery shopping and going for walks).
- Be prepared to leave housework until your return, or the next day. It can take hours to get a child with reflux ready to go out, particularly the 'vomity' ones.
- Short outings are often best (e.g. a trip to the park in the stroller).
- If you know you are going on an outing that is stressful to you, plan to reduce that stress (e.g. take an understanding person with you so you do not have to cope alone), pack bags/food the day before and change your child just before leaving (if they are a vomiter).

## Comforting Your Child

Some of the suggestions listed below may help you comfort your child. As with all suggestions, try those you feel comfortable with, as long as they are safe. Talk to your doctor if you have any concerns.

*"We were often told we'd spoil our baby if we picked her up when she cried. We decided to follow our instincts and pick her up if we felt we should, and deal with any problems later on. That was the key to our survival!"*

- Learn about infant behavioural clues; read or talk to your child-health nurse about how to communicate with your infant. Through their cues, infants tell us about how they feel, how much stimulation they can tolerate and when they need rest, sleep, play and food.

- Check to make sure your child is comfortable. Check to see that clothing, including the nappy, is not too tight, and that it is clean and dry.
- Comfort your child by holding them, especially if their reflux is causing pain. Close contact, especially skin on skin, can be very comforting for your child as well as you. Sitting or lying down to hold your child or carrying your infant around in a baby sling can really make a difference. Rocking, swaying, dancing or any other rhythmic movements can be soothing.
- Massage can be soothing to infants and children, and it can also aid digestion. Consider learning how to massage your infant or child so they get the most out of it.
- Try to comfort your child earlier, rather than later. If they have been crying for a while, they can take longer to calm down, and being distressed may cause them to reflux more. It may be easier to avert the situation and comfort your child when you can.
- If you choose to bring your infant into bed with you for comfort, ensure you follow the recommendations for reducing the risk of sudden infant death and fatal sleeping accidents. This is outlined in the SIDS and Kids Information statement entitled 'Sleeping with Baby' (available at www.sidsandkids.org).
- Give your infant a bath, or have a warm bath with them at any time of the day. It can be relaxing for both of you, and it also provides further skin-on-skin contact. Try gentle rocking backwards and forwards in the bath and

gentle strokes on their tummy. Have a support person present if bathing with your infant.

*"Harrison would often get a nice warm bath in the middle of the night. It was the only thing that would stop him screaming and then we could all get back to bed." Tania*

- Try water play (with full supervision from an adult). Water may calm children with reflux.
- Rock your infant gently in your arms or in a baby swing, hammock or rocking chair, which can help them bring up wind. Crying infants can swallow air, which can cause abdominal pain and reflux. If rocking or gentle motion is not soothing, try complete stillness and slow movements and see if that helps.

---

*Never leave your infant unattended or sleeping unsupervised in devices such as swings, hammocks, chairs and bouncinettes. These devices were not designed as infant sleep environments and many do not have Australian safety standards. Fatal accidents have occurred.*

---

- Some infants with reflux have a need to suck almost constantly. Encourage your infant to find their finger or fist to suck on, allow them to suck on your clean finger, or consider offering a dummy/pacifier.
- Provide soothing music. Sing lullabies to your child or use relaxation CDs (e.g. heartbeat or ocean sounds). Position your child on your tummy so they can hear your heartbeat.
- Provide your child with 'white noise' from a CD, radio or white-noise device. Consider using appliances in the

background (e.g. vacuum cleaner, air conditioner, fan).

- If your child starts to become unsettled, take them to a quiet, dimly lit room. This may work if you do it early.
- Know your infant's cues and respond appropriately. Some infants enjoy having their environment stimulating as it keeps them interested and distracted, while others prefer having their environment subdued.
- Feed your child if they are due to be fed – putting it off until later may upset them further.
- Try wrapping your infant as you would for sleep, and cuddle them. The principles of safe infant wrapping are outlined in the SIDS and Kids information statement entitled "Wrapping Infants" (available at www.sidsand kids.org).
- Give your child a soft toy or other small item such as a handkerchief that has your smell on it. Try wearing it inside your clothes for a while before giving it to them.
- A walk in the pram or drive in the car (if you aren't too tired) can sometimes be soothing.
- Your child may sense if you are feeling upset, angry or overwhelmed. If possible, let your partner, family member or friend care for your child while you take some time for yourself.

# 4

# Positioning Children with Reflux

## Infants and Children Under the Age of Two Years

### General Positioning Strategies

To help manage an infant's reflux, it is generally recommended that you feed them while they are as upright as possible and keep them upright for at least thirty minutes afterwards. It may also help if you hold them upright at other times as well. This is not always easy, but some infants will let you know, in no uncertain terms, that they are more comfortable that way! Additional strategies that may help are listed below.

*"The advice about keeping bub upright after feeds has helped us a lot . . . even lately when she has been really bad with asthma, eczema and reflux, holding her upright is the only way I can get her to sleep."*

- Use positions that suit your infant, providing they meet safety recommendations. Avoid positions that place unnecessary pressure on your infant's stomach e.g. seated positions, particularly after feeds.

- A baby sling/carrier that allows your infant to be upright and minimises pressure on their abdomen may be helpful in managing reflux, and may provide you with a free hand to work. Some slings can cause small infants to slump, which has the potential to obstruct their airway as well as causing more reflux, so consider experimenting with various types to find one that suits. Older infants may prefer a backpack.
- Carry your infant upright, with their head over your shoulder. This position may also be preferable when burping them, especially when they are very young, as sitting them on your lap can put pressure on their stomach.
- A rocking chair may help. It allows you to sit while holding your infant upright, and also enjoy some quiet, soothing movement.
- Avoid rough handling or bouncing. You may need to remind family and friends of this.
- Place your infant's body down your arm, with their head close to your elbow, and support them with your hand on their crotch. Hold them with their head higher than their stomach, and if necessary, you can pat your infant using your other hand (see photo).
- Use a reclining bouncinette while your infant is supervised.

*Never leave your infant to sleep in a bouncinette unsupervised. Fatal sleeping accidents have occurred when infants have been left unsupervised in bouncinettes.*

- If sitting down with your infant, place them on your lap (facing away from you) as you lean back slightly. This position can reduce pressure in the abdomen.

*"We used an [activity centre] . . . like a walker without wheels. He seemed to like these as he was upright and could move around . . . gives you a bit of a break during the day."* Karen

*"A baby swim ring helps bub sit up; if they fall over it is soft, and they may enjoy tapping their fingers on the side."* Trudi *(supervise fully)*

## Nappy Changing

Some strategies that may help with nappy changing are listed below:

- If possible, change your infant's nappy before a feed rather than after, as reflux is more likely to occur with a full tummy.
- Avoid lifting your infant's legs too high; turn them to the side for cleaning and nappy changing.
- Keep nappy loose, with as little pressure as possible on your child's stomach. Try to avoid clothes with tight elasticised waists.

## Tummy Time

> Supervision by an adult is essential when providing an infant with tummy time.

Tummy time is important for all infants as it contributes to their motor development and reduces the risk of infants developing flat spots on their head. Tummy time should be started soon after birth; schedule as many tummy-time sessions as possible each day, before feeds and while your infant is awake and alert. While some infants with reflux only tolerate tummy time for short periods initially, the key is perseverance. Most infants tolerate being on their tummies for longer as they grow older and stronger. The following suggestions may help; however, discuss any concerns you have with your doctor or child-health nurse:

- Try to make tummy time fun and stimulating, with lots of toys to amuse your infant. Lie beside or in front of them and sing or tell nursery rhymes as a distraction.

*"Lie on the floor in front of them or lie them so they're facing a mirror (they love looking in mirrors)." Nelle*

- Try tummy time on your bed instead of the floor. As always, fully supervise, and never leave your infant unattended on the bed.
- If your infant objects to being laid flat on their tummy, try using a reflux wedge. Never leave your infant unattended, or allow them to sleep on the wedge.
- Lie on your back and place your infant on your chest, tummy to tummy, facing you. It may help them feel more secure to be in this position, and it may also distract them.
- Tummy time can be fun if you try different positions (e.g. put your infant on their tummy for massage, or support them on an exercise ball or in the bath). Alternatively, you could sit on a chair with your infant lying on your lap.

*"I put my daughter on a blow-up water mat that encourages tummy time . . . it was soft underneath and she enjoyed watching things move." Tania*

## Positioning for Sleep
*By Professor (Adjunct) Jeanine Young,*
*Nursing Director – Research*
Always follow the SIDS and Kids Safe Sleeping recommenda-

tions for positioning your infant for sleep. To sleep them safely and reduce the risk of sudden infant death:

- Sleep your infant on their back from birth, never on their tummy or side.
- Sleep your infant with their head and face uncovered.
- Avoid exposing your infant to cigarette smoke, before and after birth.
- Sleep your infant in their own cot or bassinette in the same room as you for their first six to twelve months.
- Provide a safe sleeping environment, night and day: safe cot, safe mattress, safe bedding and safe sleeping place.
  - Put your infant's feet at the bottom of the cot.
  - The cot must meet the Australian standard for cots.
  - No additional mattresses or extra padding should be placed in a travel cot.
  - Tuck in bedclothes securely so bedding is not loose.
  - Keep quilts, doonas, duvets, pillows, cot bumpers, sheepskins and soft toys out of the cot or sleeping place.
  - Use a firm, clean mattress that fits snugly in the cot.
  - Bouncinettes, hammocks, prams and strollers have not been designed as sleeping products and your infant should not be left unsupervised if they fall asleep in them.

You may be concerned about sleeping your infant on their back; however, this position does not increase their risk of breathing in or choking on their milk or vomit. Infants with reflux should be placed on their back to sleep on a firm, flat mattress that is not elevated. Healthy infants protect their airway when placed supine (on their back), as long as their swallowing and arousal abilities are not impaired.

Side positioning is unstable and not recommended as an alternative to sleeping your infant on their back. Aids and devices intended to keep infants in certain sleep positions are not recommended; they do not prevent your infant from rolling onto their tummy (prone), and they limit their movements as they get older.

As infants grow older, beyond the age of five to six months, a safe cot and safe sleep environment is still necessary even though they will move around the cot and roll over. Settle your infant to sleep on their back, but let them find the sleep position they feel most comfortable in.

Parents of some infants with a rare medical condition may be advised by their doctor to sleep them on their left side or tummy, but only do so if your infant's doctor advises you in writing.

*The recommendations in 'Positioning for Sleep' in infants and children under the age of two years are used with permission from the Queensland Health: Safe Infant Care to Reduce the Risk of Sudden Unexpected Deaths in Infancy Policy and Guidelines (2008), which is consistent with SIDS and Kids (2009) and the Public Health Association of Australia (2008) guidelines.*

## Children Over the Age of Two Years and Teenagers

### Positioning for Sleep

Children in this age group will find the sleep position they feel most comfortable in. However, they may find lying on their tummy or left side more comfortable because these positions may reduce reflux episodes. These positions are not recommended for children under twelve months of age, when they are at increased risk for sudden infant death.

Some children over the age of one or two years may also find it more comfortable with the head of their bed elevated by thirty degrees. Bricks may be placed under the bedposts at the head of the bed to raise it ten to twenty centimetres. If this does not help, consider altering the angle or see if they sleep better with the bed flat.

Other strategies that may be helpful are similar to those suggestions for infants (e.g. staying upright after feeds and avoiding lying down for two to three hours). As with all reflux treatments, it may be a matter of trial and error to find what works best, but if there are ever any concerns, you or your teenager should discuss them with a health professional.

# 5

# General Information
# on Sleeping

As with all suggestions, try those you feel happy with and feel are appropriate, as long as these strategies are safe. If it works and you are happy to continue with it, that is fine. If not, try something else. Always follow the SIDS and Kids Safe Sleeping guidelines, and if you are concerned about any aspect of your child's sleeping, or other issues, please discuss this with your doctor or child-health nurse.

## Sleeping Issues

Sleeping issues, as outlined in earlier chapters, are frequently encountered in infants and children, but when an infant or child suffers from reflux, these issues can be even more difficult to control. If your child suffers from sleeping issues they may be tired, irritable and difficult to manage, and they may have issues when settling or with restless, easily disturbed sleep. They may object to lying down, particularly after a feed. They may take short naps during the day and may wake in a distressed state.

They may also wake frequently overnight. Even if your child does sleep all night, as some children with reflux do, they can still be difficult to manage when they are awake.

If your sleep is being disturbed regularly, you may be exhausted. This can make it harder for you to care for your child, and can also affect how you interact with other family members. When stress and concern for your child is added in, these sleep issues can be even more complex, confusing and difficult to overcome.

Also, it is often hard to know what is caused by reflux and what is behavioural. If your child objects to being laid down to sleep, are they more comfortable in an upright position, or do they want to be held? On top of that, there are many conflicting pieces of advice regarding sleep and settling management for children, from attachment parenting and sharing the bed, to controlled comforting and settling infants on their own.

Some strategies are not always appropriate for your child when they have reflux – you may worry that your child is uncomfortable, or you may not be able to use controlled-comforting strategies if your child vomits when they become distressed. However, there is no reason why you cannot try safe settling techniques if you feel comfortable with them, and if you feel they are right for your child and the situation. Remember that just because your child has reflux, it does not mean they cannot learn to sleep better, though you may need to be more flexible with trying various safe techniques. On the other hand, if you feel that the reflux is the reason for your child's continuing sleep issues, then comforting them may be appropriate. It can be a matter of doing what works, and if that is the only way you can get your child to sleep (at least temporarily), and it is safe, it may be what you need to do.

*"I have a school-aged son so the textbooks don't work when [babies] just fall asleep and you have to [go] out again . . . I [also] don't have the time to stand there for twenty minutes patting him on the back . . . the nurse in the mother/baby unit . . . said you need to do whatever works to get him through the pain . . . she said that we will probably end up with sleeping issues but we could address that later when the reflux was sorted and that's pretty much what we've done." Kylie W*

If your child continues to have sleep difficulties, either falling asleep or staying asleep, it may mean that reflux is still an issue and a review by a child-health nurse or doctor may be advised.

Until any sleep issues improve, it may help if you do not watch the time or calculate how much sleep you missed. Knowing how much sleep you are missing out on can make you feel worse by making you feel more tense and exhausted, and can also affect your child.

## Suggestions for Settling Infants and Children Under the Age of Two Years

As with other aspects of parenting, settling techniques are often trial and error and what works at one age may not work at another. If you are not comfortable with an idea, try something else, or discuss it with your doctor first. Remember to always follow the SIDS and Kids Safe Sleeping public health recommendations for infants.

The following settling techniques that have been suggested are aimed primarily at infants, but many can also be adapted for other age groups as well. *For information on positioning for sleep, refer to previous chapter.*

- Watch for signs of tiredness and pick the right time to put your child to bed. Depending on their age, you may notice signs like jerky limb movements, clenched fists, yawning, irritability or eye rubbing. Talk to your child-health nurse if you are not sure what signs to look for.
- Try giving your child a massage, particularly if they are unsettled. This may help relax them enough so they can sleep.
- Establish a bedtime ritual (e.g. bath, quiet playtime, feed), ensuring they are held upright for half an hour following it, a few bedtime stories, and then to bed so your infant knows what to expect.
- If you are comfortable considering this, try offering your infant a dummy at all sleep times – some find the sucking action soothing.
- Carry your infant around in a sling during the day. Being close to you, and able to listen to your heartbeat, can help them relax and sleep.
- Experiment with tucking your infant's sheets in. This can be done if your infant is wrapped; however, take care to ensure bedding type and amount used follows safe-sleeping recommendations, so your infant's head remains uncovered and they do not get too hot. Some infants settle as they appear to find being tucked in comforting.
- Try not to feed your child too close to bedtime as this may cause them to reflux.
- If your child is on reflux medication it may help to give these as close to bedtime as possible. It may be possible to make it part of the bedtime routine. Check with your pharmacist or doctor to ensure this timing for medication is suitable for your child's needs.

- Observe your child's habits and determine if the amount of sleep they have during the day affects their sleep patterns at night.
- Concentrate on getting a good feeding routine established as this can help with establishing sleeping routines.
- Leave something that has your smell in your infant's bed (e.g. a breast pad if breastfeeding as it is small). The smell may help some sensitive infants settle.
- Encourage and allow your partner to share in the nighttime parenting.
- Infants with reflux can be very sensitive to noise and may wake very easily, so using white noise may be helpful (e.g. air-conditioner, radio, CD with music or lullabies), or repetitive noise like a vacuum cleaner or washing machine. Avoid unnecessary noise/stimuli – make sure all door hinges are oiled, and floorboards do not creak.
- Some children with reflux do better if you hold them until they are deeply asleep, while others are better if you put them to bed when they are drowsy but not asleep.
- Dress your child appropriately for the weather (rather than adding extra blankets), so they are comfortable enough to be able to sleep.
- Try having a light on. If this does not work, try turning it off or dimming it.
- Try using a rocking chair; movement can relax your child.
- Try putting your infant to sleep in a baby rocker while wrapped, and once sound asleep, try moving your infant to their bed. Ensure they are not left in this unsafe sleeping environment; your infant should be supervised at all times when they are placed in an environment not designed for infant sleep.

- If your infant does not seem to be settling, consider taking them for a walk in their pram, giving a massage or relaxing bath and then trying to settle again.
- Comfort your child as necessary; any sleep-training methods that encourage you to let your child 'cry it out' may not necessarily be appropriate for a child with reflux.
- Caffeine can increase the number of reflux episodes and impact on sleep. If breastfeeding, minimise the amount of caffeine you consume as it can pass through your breastmilk, and older children should also avoid or minimise caffeine.

## Additional Settling Suggestions
*By Professor (Adjunct) Jeanine Young,*
*Nursing Director – Research*

- Experiment with infant wrapping techniques – they are effective sleep and settling strategies for infants until four to six months of age. Wrapping can reduce crying time and episodes of waking, and may also help to keep your infant in the recommended back position. Always follow safe wrapping principles:
  - Ensure your infant is positioned on their back with feet at the bottom of the cot.
  - Ensure your infant's head is not covered, and there are no doonas, cot bumpers or soft toys in the cot.
  - Wrap your infant firmly but not tightly.
  - Use lightweight cotton or muslin material and ensure your infant is not overdressed under the wrap.
  - Never position your infant on their tummy when wrapped.
  - Never wrap your infant if they are sharing a sleep surface with another person.

- Try a variety of wrapping techniques to find one that suits your infant best (e.g. arms inside wrap, one or both arms/hands out, hands near mouth).
- Modify the wrap to meet the baby's developmental changes (e.g. arms free once startle reflex begins to disappear at around three months; Moro or startle reflex should have disappeared by four to five months).
- When baby is able to roll from their back to their tummy and then onto their back again during supervised play (usually four to six months) the use of a wrap can be discontinued for settling and sleep. The wrap may prevent an older infant who has turned onto their tummy during sleep from returning to the back-sleeping position.
- For more information see the SIDS and Kids information statement of wrapping infants, available at www.sidsandkids.org.

• Consider using a safe-infant sleeping bag for your infant. Many infants with reflux are very restless sleepers, and this eliminates the need to continually check that your infant's body is covered while their head and face remains uncovered. These sleeping bags are the correct size for your infant, with fitted neck, arm holes or sleeves and no hood.

• It is acknowledged that many parents choose to bring their infant into bed with them for feeding or settling. Sharing sleep may work for some families; however, safety guidelines must be strictly followed to reduce the risk of sudden infant death or fatal sleeping accidents. For more information, see the SIDS and Kids information statement on 'Sleeping with a baby' available at www.sidsandkids.org. Bedding must be arranged so it cannot cover your infant's face; and you must ensure your infant cannot fall out of bed. SIDS and Kids suggest that sidecar cots may be an alternative, as they attach to your bed and provide closeness while providing a separate sleeping surface for your infant.

- It is not safe to share a sleep surface with your infant if either you or your partner are smokers, under the influence of alcohol or drugs that cause sedation, or excessively tired.

• Your infant must never be left alone on an adult bed or put to sleep on a sofa, bean bag, waterbed or sagging mattress.

• If you are comfortable considering this, letting your infant sleep upright on your chest can be helpful. Avoid falling asleep with your infant while on a sofa because this increases the risk of sudden unexpected death in infancy. While this may be difficult due to exhaustion, it is important you are aware of this and you put your infant back to bed before you fall asleep on the sofa.

• Infants born prematurely are known to be more likely to experience reflux; they may also experience difficulty settling as their early development has been affected by an environment in the neonatal unit that is full of stimuli – noise, smells, touch, positioning and so on. Be aware of your infant's individual needs when choosing settling strategies.

*The strategies in 'Additional Settling Suggestions' were written by Dr Jeanine Young (used with her permission, 4/2/10) and are consistent with current SIDS and Kids guidelines. Guidelines on infant wrapping and other topics are available at SIDS and Kids (www.sidsandkids.org).*

## If Your Child Wakes

Some of the following suggestions may be useful if your child wakes:

- Check your child's comfort level: are they too hot or cold; do they need a feed; does their nappy need changing? Attend to these needs as necessary.

- Is your child actively refluxing or in pain? If so, attend to this sooner rather than later. Holding your child upright may help their reflux settle. Trust your instincts and comfort your child as you feel is right.

- Once you are satisfied your child is comfortable, begin the process of settling again, while respecting their need for comfort.

- Limit any interaction with your child when they are awake during the night (e.g. avoid eye contact and talking, and keep lighting as low as possible).

- Try to reduce night feeds if they are no longer necessary. Talk to your doctor if you are unsure, especially if your infant's weight gain is an issue.

# 6

# General Information on Feeding

## Breast and Formula Feeding

Feeding issues are common in children with reflux, whether they are breastfed, formula-fed or on solids, and children may be very demanding and difficult to feed. Some of these issues may be easily corrected with simple strategies, but others may not be, and feeds and mealtimes can sometimes be a major source of concern and frustration.

> *"Having a baby struggle to feed is exhausting. Instead of having that loving quiet time while your baby snuggles in and breast-feeds beautifully, you've got a baby who is fighting you and your breast. Some mums feel that their baby is rejecting them, even while knowing on some level that this isn't the case. While it's not unreasonable to look for a more 'normal' feeding relationship with your baby, you may find it's really the reflux that is the problem, not the method of feeding."*

Despite any difficulties, your concerns may be dismissed and you may hear statements such as "no child will starve themselves", or "they will eat when they are hungry". This is not necessarily true when your child has reflux, no matter what age they are, and you may instinctively realise this. You may blame yourself (or others may blame you) for all the issues, you may be concerned about the milk causing problems and you may agonise over how you should feed your child. You may wonder if you should give up breastfeeding, or change to another formula. Others may pressure you to stop breastfeeding in favour of thickened formula, and if you are formula feeding you may be pressured about not breastfeeding.

*"I was told that there was something wrong with my milk or I didn't have enough because my daughter cried when I fed her. Of course I thought it was my fault!"*

No matter what the issues are, it is important you know you are not alone and that the issues are not your fault. If you are breastfeeding, there is no indication for you to stop. Reflux occurs in both breast and formula fed infants, and for most infants, breastfeeding is still the recommended option. There are no guarantees that switching from breastmilk to formula, or changing formula, will improve your child's reflux or feeding behaviours in any way.

*"At seven weeks, in desperation, I gave up breastfeeding, hoping that bottles would keep him full for longer and that he could feed in a more upright position. None of that worked and we just became more tired and anxious."* Nelle

When you have the additional pressure of dealing with reflux, it is important you gain support and understanding regardless of how you feed your child. It may help to try some of the suggestions provided in this chapter if they seem appropriate for your situation. However, if your child continues to suffer from feeding issues or they are causing a lot of distress, it is important you seek medical advice and address the issues early.

## Breastfeeding

Breastfeeding is the 'biologically normal' way to feed an infant and the majority of mothers should be encouraged to breast-feed, despite the difficulties of reflux. Breastmilk is the most complete form of nutrition for normal growth and development of infants. It also provides your infant protection against many diseases and infections, and the cost of breastfeeding is small compared to the considerable cost of using formula.

Breastmilk is more easily digested and empties more rapidly from the stomach than infant formula, so it makes sense that if an infant refluxes on breastmilk they can also reflux on infant formula. It has also been shown that breastfed infants have much shorter reflux episodes during sleep compared to formula-fed infants. Additionally, regurgitated breastmilk may not be as irritating to the oesophagus as regurgitated infant formula, and breastmilk contains substances that can help repair the lining of the oesophagus.

Breastfeeding also has practical advantages compared to formula feeding. It is more convenient, with no preparation, clean-up or sterilisation required, and it always provides feeds at the right temperature. It involves no guesswork to figure out how many bottles to make up or how much formula to put in them. This can make breastfeeding especially helpful as infants with reflux may take some feeds well whilst they fuss or fight at others. Breastfeeding also releases hormones that can help a mother cope with an unsettled infant.

If you are breastfeeding, you may need continued support and guidance because of the difficult circumstances reflux can bring. If you have any questions or concerns about feeding issues, for example milk supply, breast refusal or pain with breastfeeding, it may help to speak to a child-health nurse, lactation consultant, breastfeeding counsellor, or speech pathologist who has experience dealing with children's feeding issues.

It is also worth mentioning that feeding your infant expressed breastmilk may be an option if breastfeeding is not possible or you need a break. Others can participate in the feeds, and your infant can still reap the benefits from breastmilk.

## Formula Feeding

It is recognised that your infant may be formula-fed for a variety of reasons, whether it is a decision you made voluntarily or was forced upon you.

> *"I'm really hoping not to go down the formula track, although [the doctors] said . . . it may be necessary for medical reasons . . . all reflux parents will do whatever they need to make their child better, so if that means formula for us, then so be it."*

If you are formula feeding or considering it, it is important you know that formula fed infants can and do thrive. Commercial infant formulas are breastmilk substitutes designed to closely match the composition of breastmilk. Additionally, formula fed infants do not need to miss out on the closeness provided by breastfeeding, and you still have opportunities to cuddle your infant whilst feeding.

There can also be some advantages to formula feeding an infant with reflux. Foremost, it can relieve some of the stress on you, particularly if you are not coping or receiving enough support.

If you want to try formula feeding, it may help if you maintain your supply of breastmilk so you can return to breastfeeding if you choose/prefer to. Be aware that many infants show improvement in the first few days or weeks on changing to bottle feeding, but this is sometimes only temporary.

For information on feeding your infant with formula, or if you have any questions or concerns, speak to a child-health nurse, dietitian or speech pathologist. A speech pathologist who has experience dealing with children's feeding issues can help you with flow rates, sucking and pacing issues, and can help you choose an appropriate teat for your infant.

## Feeding Difficulties in Breast and Bottle Fed Infants

Your infant may develop a variety of difficult feeding behaviours because of reflux, and it may also be difficult for them to put on weight. They may associate feeding with the pain or other discomfort they feel, or they may not develop necessary skills for eating because of their reflux. They may then refuse to feed and may turn their head away and cry even before the feed begins, sometimes as soon as they see the breast or bottle, and may gag and vomit as well. Alternatively, they may fuss throughout the entire feed or they may take a small amount of the feed without difficulty, and then cry and pull away. If their aversion is severe enough they may only accept feeds while they are asleep or drowsy (sometimes referred to as 'dream feeds').

> *"Jorja isn't feeding well . . . I was feeding standing up rocking her but now she just attaches, has five sucks, cries then tries to go on again. I've resorted to a syringe with [expressed breastmilk] though sometimes she feeds while she's sleepy." Trudi*

If your infant has feeding issues, it may be difficult for you or your infant to enjoy feeds, and you may find yourself trying different strategies to get them to eat. (In some cases, the association between feeding and pain is so ingrained that even if the pain is controlled they may not realise the feeding experience will be any different.) If feeding issues are causing concerns, then your child may benefit from an assessment from a speech pathologist who has feeding experience in infants and toddlers, and/or a dietitian.

*"I sought help from a speech pathologist with Lara, and she gave us tips to help with bottle-feeding. My sister-in-law also recently took her baby to one, and she was able to help her choose a bottle that was more suitable to her baby." Tania*

Be aware that other conditions can cause feeding difficulties. If your infant suddenly starts to refuse to feed or you notice any other difficulties, talk to your doctor.

## Strategies for Feeding Difficulties

There may be strategies you can try, no matter what the issues are. If one does not work, consider trying the opposite, so long as it is safe. You never know what will help, but if you do find something, stick with it! Talk to your doctor if you are concerned for any reason.

Some suggestions that may help with feeding difficulties have been listed here. These suggestions have been provided by parents of children who have reflux:

- Prepare yourself mentally and physically before a feed.
  - Take a few deep breaths or use other relaxation tech-

niques so you can relax as much as possible. Tension can make your infant feel tense also.

- Try letting someone else calm your infant while you calm yourself. When you are both ready, take a few seconds to prepare, and think positive thoughts.
- Arrange a comfortable spot to feed and eliminate possible interruptions (e.g. occupy older siblings with activities, divert the phone).
- Put on some soothing music (e.g. relaxation CD).
- Visualise your infant feeding. This can help you relax, which can help them relax.
- Watch your self-talk; try not to think about how long your infant has had feeding issues or how long they may continue. Try to focus on the moment.
- Remind yourself that this is not the most important feed of your infant's life. If this one is not successful, there is always next time.
- Try to accept frustration as a temporary 'norm'.
- Resist the temptation to compare your infant with others; every infant is different and should be treated individually.
- If possible, concentrate on feeds when your partner is home or a friend is available so they can occupy any toddlers.
- If your infant is refusing feeds, try to keep perspective. How many times are they totally refusing? If your infant is older, can they go longer between feeds?
• Comfort is important for your infant to feed well. If your infant is screaming, hiccupping, seems to be in pain or obviously refluxing, wait until they have settled.
• Try to keep your infant in an upright position while feed-

ing and for thirty minutes after; keep their body straight and avoid slumping. If they are less likely to reflux during the feed, they may feel more comfortable and may feed better. Additionally, their stomach may empty faster, which can mean they reflux less.

- Try getting your infant into a routine (if possible).
- Consider feeding your infant while you are in a hammock or rocking chair, or while they are in a baby sling.
- Try feeding your infant smaller amounts more frequently (this should not be more often than every three hours). If their stomach is not full, there may be less pressure on their lower oesophageal sphincter and they may reflux less. However, this does not suit all infants. If your infant is not satisfied or becomes distressed with smaller feeds, consider giving larger amounts with a longer time between feeds.
- Try massaging your infant before a feed; this can help them relax as well as aid digestion.
- Do not rush the feed; keep it calm and quiet. If that does not work, try feeding more quickly.
- Try to minimise the amount of air your infant swallows during a feed. This may depend on them getting a good seal on the breast or bottle. There are some specially designed bottles and teats on the market that may help.
- Burp your infant throughout the feed, but do not interrupt if they are feeding comfortably. Experiment with how often; a breastfed infant may swallow less air than a bottle-fed infant, and an older infant may not need to be burped as often.
- Do not try to force your infant to feed if they are fussing, continually refusing or not interested in the feed, as this

can make the issue worse. Wait fifteen to thirty minutes and try again (e.g. they may not want a feed at 5.30 am, but when offered thirty minutes later may feed well). In the meantime, use distractions to try and settle them.

- If your infant is refusing feeds and is on solids, try adding lots of their milk (prepared infant formula or breastmilk) to rice cereal, or use thickener to make custard or blancmange.

*"[I make] custard and iceblocks from his formula, and add formula to his porridge." Tania*

- Aim to keep feeds no longer than twenty minutes. If feed times are regularly longer than this, seek guidance from a lactation consultant or paediatric feeding speech pathologist.
- It may help to avoid distractions while feeding your infant. Feed in a quiet, darkened room, keep noise to a minimum (talking may disturb some infants) and try to refrain from annoying disturbances such as tickling their feet. Alternatively, if your infant feeds better when distracted, try using a baby's mobile, the television, or attach toys to your clothes. Try using distractions if you notice they are about to reflux.
- Consider having soft music or some steady noise (e.g. vacuum cleaner in the background).
- Feed your infant when they are due for a feed, and before they get desperately hungry. Look for feeding cues such as bringing their hands up to their mouth. Ideally, feeding should start before your infant is crying for food.
- Do not feed your infant again if they vomit; wait until the next feed to avoid overfeeding. Talk to your child

health nurse to ensure they are gaining appropriate weight.

- A play/sleep/feed routine may work better for reflux infants, but you may need to be flexible. If this does not work, consider doing the opposite.
- If your child wants to play, wait to feed them.
- If your infant has had their feed and wants to play, do not jostle them or play vigorously with them. Try to keep them upright for thirty minutes.
- If your infant is a poor sleeper, avoid feeding close to the night bedtime. If this does not work, try feeding them closer to the night sleep and see if it helps.
- Even if your infant is tired after a feed and needs to sleep, it may still help to keep them upright for thirty minutes before putting them to bed. Keep stimulation to a minimum.
- Try feeding whilst standing, and rock gently; make soothing noises such as humming, 'ssh-ing' or singing. Make any monotonous rhythmical pattern.
- Try repositioning yourself with a minimum of movement in your infant. Some infants will not return to feeding if they have been disturbed.
- If you are comfortable with the idea, consider using a dummy; place it in, take it out and quickly replace with breast, teat or spoonful of solids. Do not rely on it for too long as it may tire some infants so they refuse to feed.
- Cuddle your infant or distract them with physical contact or doing something different (e.g. a walk outdoors). When they are settled, try to ease them onto the breast or bottle.
- Consider feeding your infant while you are both in a

warm bath; it is easier to clean up if they vomit. Two people may be needed to ensure your infant's safety and to help you both get out of the bath.

- Concentrate on feeds when your infant is less distressed/more relaxed as they may feed better. This may be when they are dozing off, or when stirring and not yet upset. Try to anticipate waking time and offer their feed immediately. Avoid or postpone nappy changes or turning on lights.

*"Jorja refused to feed for a month and I could only feed at night when she was asleep . . . [what] helped the most was to assume she was teething and give her ice wrapped in a cloth to suck on first." Trudi*

- If your infant is older than six months, consider offering the occasional feed in a cup. Infants do need to suck, but trying this occasionally may help. (Be aware that infants do not have the physical ability to manage cup drinking until they can coordinate breathing and swallowing, and their tongue, jaw and lip muscles are developed. Attempting to cup-feed before they have these skills may result in the milk going down into their lungs rather than their stomach.)
- Try completely different feeding positions for both you and your infant (e.g. lying on the bed with them next to you, with no body contact). This is especially good if your infant is sensing your tension. Feeding lying down may help reduce distractions (and is restful too). Position your infant upright immediately after the feed.
- Try playing with your infant on the floor and after a while, gradually offer the feed (if breastfeeding, it may

help to play with your infant while you are bare from the waist up).

- Try providing lots of skin-on-skin contact (with no pressure to feed). This may be comforting for your infant and may encourage them to feed.
- Positions that may help:
  - Hold your infant in the nursing position in your lap, but recline back so you can keep their body straight.
  - Use a reflux wedge or feeding pillow to support your infant as you feed them.
  - Stand up to feed them and cradle their body downwards (or diagonally if they are more comfortable). Try walking or rocking on your feet; if you are breastfeeding you may have to hold their head on your breast.
  - Use a baby carrier that keeps your infant upright so they can feed as you walk around. Position them so they can feed comfortably – adjust the straps to suit.
- Hold your infant close while you feed them. Chatting to them while you do this can be comforting as well as helping with their development.

## Additional Tips for Breastfeeding
- If your infant gets too frustrated before the milk flow starts, try expressing before the feed. Your infant may swallow less air if your milk has already let down.
- If you have a strong or overactive letdown (i.e. your infant is unable to keep up with the flow and gags) it may help to express milk prior to the feed so they do not have to cope with a fast flow. Alternatively, slow the flow down by nursing your infant while they are lying on top of you. Reposition them upright once the feed is established.

- If your infant is very hungry give thirty millilitres of expressed breastmilk; replace quickly with your breast (after the letdown). This may help infants who do not like to suck for too long, and may prevent them from choking or gulping, which can upset a child with reflux.

*"I would try and express off about twenty to thirty millilitres BEFORE a feed . . . [to] get more hind milk this way."* Shell

- Concentrate on feeds when your milk supply is at its peak (e.g. during the night or early morning).
- You may like to experiment with feeding from one or both breasts to see what suits your infant best. Some are better if they are offered both breasts, while others are better if they are offered only one breast each feed.
- If you offer both breasts in a feed, keep your infant in the same position and gently move them over, rather than turning them around.
- Encourage your infant to rest against your bare breast between feeds (without trying to feed) so the pain of feeding is not associated with contact with your skin or breast.
- Try feeding in the twins' position/football hold (with your infant's body under your arm, angled downward to keep their head higher than their stomach).

*"I found the football hold . . . helps as their head and necks are in a more upright position than [when] lying across your body."* Shell

- Try sitting your infant beside you on the chair, facing towards your breast. Ensure their head is slightly higher than your nipple (see photo).

- Try feeding your infant while you recline on a bed (arrange pillows) or in a reclining chair.
- If your infant is older, sit them on your lap or try straddling their legs around your hips.

## Additional Tips for Bottle Feeding

- Do not screw the teat on too tightly, thus preventing air bubbles from escaping.
- Do not force your infant to finish the bottle – a distended stomach may cause more reflux.
- Experiment with different teats and bottles to find ones that suit your infant. Be aware that more expensive is not necessarily better. Some bottles are angled, which may help with upright feeding, while others are designed to eliminate air bubbles and reduce wind. A child-health nurse or a speech pathologist who specialises in feeding issues may be able to help.
- Try gently tickling your infant's lips with the teat, rather than forcing it into their mouth. Your infant may then be more willing to accept the bottle.
- Try sitting your infant in a reclining position, e.g. sit your infant in your lap facing outwards and lean back (see photo), or sit them in a bouncinette or high chair. Once the feed is finished, hold your infant upright as much as possible.

## Comfort Feeding

Infants sometimes want to comfort feed because of their reflux, and some put on a lot of weight as a result. These infants seem to work out it is soothing when they feed and may constantly demand or look for a feed. This can mean they tend to 'graze' a lot rather than having a proper feed. They may not be hungry but may simply be trying to feel more comfortable.

Some of these infants guzzle their feeds, and can be desperate to drink more. Others may be entirely different, and may combine the need to feed frequently with pulling off and fighting at the breast or bottle.

A medical study has shown that about three-quarters of all reflux episodes occur either during the feed, or within the first two hours of a feed, which correlates with a child demanding to be fed in that time frame. Unfortunately, this can set up a cycle because frequent feeds (e.g. one to two hourly) means your child may be frequently refluxing the entire time. If they learn to feed to momentarily soothe the pain, their stomach has less opportunity to empty and may overfill, which may increase their chance of refluxing. Their solution may be to look for another feed so they feel better, which can set up the whole process again.

## Strategies for Comfort Feeding

While some of the previously listed strategies may help if your child is trying to feed too frequently, i.e. feeding for comfort rather than nutritional needs, these additional strategies (provided by parents who have children with reflux) may also help.

- It is important to differentiate between the need for a cuddle and hunger cues; you could try other comfort measures before offering the breast/bottle.
- Try to gradually increase times between feeds, rather than change feeding times drastically. Check weight gain with your child-health nurse or doctor to ensure their growth is adequate. Also be aware that infants go through growth spurts and will want to feed more during these

times. Keep a diary so you can keep track of feed times and the number of feeds, and review it each week (not daily).

- Try to distract your infant from a feed and comfort them in other ways. Change their environment (go for a walk, offer stimulating toys), or try to keep them amused.
- If you are breastfeeding, enlist the help of others so your infant is not close to you and cannot smell their next feed.
- Consider offering a dummy, your clean finger or a bottle of water for your infant to suck on instead of offering a feed.
- If advised by your doctor, administer an antacid or other prescribed medication as your infant may be demanding a feed as a way to soothe pain. This may help them feed better and it can help delay the time until their feed is due.
- If breastfeeding, try one-sided feeding so they receive more hind milk, as it has more fat and kilojoules than foremilk. Your infant may feel fuller for longer with less volume, which may mean they reflux less.
- It is important you do not overfeed your infant as this is likely to contribute to their reflux and their discomfort. So you know how much to put in each bottle (if bottle-feeding), work out the volume your infant needs over twenty-four hours and divide by the number of feeds they have each day.

## Thickened Feeds/Food Thickeners

Thickened feeds/thickening agents are often recommended for infants as a way of treating reflux as they are believed to be more difficult to reflux than liquids. Some infants respond extremely well to food thickeners though others do not, and some infants become more unsettled. While studies have shown mixed results, it seems that food thickeners can reduce the amount and frequency of vomiting in some children, but do not reduce the amount of time the oesophagus is exposed to acid. Thickeners may increase reflux in some infants. They may also cause some infants to cough more during feeding, and diarrhoea or constipation can sometimes be a concern.

> *"I found [thickener] really helpful in controlling [my son's] vomiting. He does still vomit . . . but not as often and usually only small amounts . . . I really believe if I hadn't used it he would be very underweight."*

> *"My daughter's vomiting decreased when we stopped adding thickener in her bottle . . . the thing that was supposed to help the vomiting was actually making it worse." Tania*

If you are considering introducing thickeners to your infant, please discuss this with your doctor first. If you do introduce them, take note if the thickener seems to reduce discomfort or pain in your infant and talk to your doctor if you have any concerns. Make sure the only change you make is to thicken the milk, using a thickener designed for that purpose. Do not change formulas or amounts so you know the effect of the thickener only.

Commercial thickening agents (such as Karicare Food Thickener® or Guarcol®) are the preferred way of thickening food. They are designed to thicken milk only and generally do not change its flavour. They can be mixed with a small amount of expressed breastmilk, water or infant formula (using manufacturer's instructions) and fed to your infant as a gel before, during or after the feed.

*"Thickeners work on the principle that the heavier milk will stay in the stomach, but sometimes it sits in the throat and burns even more." Trudi*

Thickeners can also be added directly to expressed breastmilk or prepared infant formula to thicken the feed itself. This allows you the flexibility to test slightly different thicknesses until you find what best suits your infant. They can also increase the amount of kilojoules, which may suit some infants; others may drink less as a result. Infant Gaviscon® acts as a medicated thickener and may also be recommended by your doctor. Please note that Infant Gaviscon® should not be used in conjunction with other thickeners without specific medical advice.

Household foods such as rice cereal and cornflour are not recommended as thickening agents, especially for infants less than six months of age. They are better thought of as foods, and introduced when they would be used as foods. They are less convenient and more likely to be allergenic than commercial thickening agents, and if cooked, heat sensitive vitamins in the infants' milk may be destroyed. If rice cereal is used for infants over six months, it may help to start with one teaspoon per thirty millilitres of formula, and increase as tolerated to three teaspoons per thirty millilitres of formula.

Commercial AR (anti-regurgitation) formulas are already thickened. They generally have the same number of kilojoules as other infant formulas. Some infants respond better to one brand than another because of the variety of thickeners used by manufacturers. AR formulas do not allow flexibility; the thickness cannot be altered because they must be made to the correct strength. Although this suits some infants, it does not suit others.

A fast-flow (or cross-cut) teat may be more suitable for getting the thickened formula through – you may need to experiment until you find one that suits. It may also help to loosen the bottle cap or enlarge the slit to allow the milk to flow more freely.

## Feeding Issues in Children on Solids

As with younger infants, children may exhibit a variety of difficult feeding behaviours. They may accept only a few bites of food before refusing, they may totally refuse to eat solids, or may struggle with or avoid certain textures. Your child may not be able to tolerate anything other than purees, and if you try to introduce other textures they may gag, cough or vomit. On the other hand, your child may be less sensitive (hyposensitive); they may not chew their food well, and may stuff their mouth full of food. Alternatively, your child may demand food frequently (similar to an infant who comfort feeds).

> *"Anthony constantly told me he was hungry, yet would only take a few bites before wandering off, telling me he was full. I don't think he knew what hungry meant!" Glenda*

If the feeding issues are causing concerns, your child may benefit from an assessment from a dietitian and/or speech pathologist who has paediatric feeding experience. Be aware that other conditions can cause feeding difficulties, and these may need to be addressed. It is important to talk to your doctor so they can determine the cause, and also make sure there are no other factors (e.g. ear infection, enlarged tonsils), affecting your child. Your doctor can also refer your child to other services or specialists if necessary.

# General Management Strategies for Giving Solids

These suggestions have been provided by families of children with reflux. Most have been written with younger children in mind; however, some of the strategies can be adapted for older children as well. Try as many of these suggestions as you are comfortable with to find the ones that work (keep in mind that some may work one day, but not another). If you have concerns or your child is having difficulties, seek advice from your doctor, child-health nurse, dietitian or speech pathologist who specialises in children with feeding issues:

- Around four to six months your infant may show signs of being ready to start solids (e.g. being interested in food eaten by others). Read, or talk to your child-health nurse, about how to recognise these signs.
- Solids and posture go hand in hand. Find the best position for your infant when giving solids (e.g. sitting in your lap or in a high chair). A reclining position may work best, but be careful they are not in a position that increases the pressure on their tummy, i.e. slumped.
  - Your child may prefer a different position for different feeds or on different days, depending on how bad their reflux is at the time.
- Hold your infant upright after solids to help minimise reflux and help them burp. Handling them with extreme care can make the difference between a calm or screaming infant.
- Try to avoid overfeeding. If your child vomits what seems to be all their meal immediately after eating, they may not want or need to eat again straight away. Talk to your child-health nurse if you are unsure how much they should be eating for their age and weight.

- Encourage your child to eat smaller meals more frequently.
- Avoid or minimise foods if they seem to cause irritation or increase the risk of reflux. If these foods do not seem to cause discomfort or other difficulties, it may not be necessary to limit them. If you are unsure, seek advice from a child health nurse, doctor or dietitian.
  - Spicy foods, citrus fruits (e.g. oranges, grapefruit and their juices), tomatoes and other acidic food, carbonated drinks, and peppermint and spearmint oils can be irritating, and omission of these from the diet can sometimes be helpful.
  - Fatty foods (e.g. chocolate, fried foods, cream, animal/vegetable oils) can decrease the efficiency of the lower oesophageal sphincter or slow the rate the stomach empties. *"Be aware of this; and watch the amount of fat or oil your child can manage." Joan Breakey, dietitian*
  - Caffeine can relax the lower oesophageal sphincter, increase the amount of stomach acid secreted, and increase the risk of GORD. It can also impact on sleep and can cause irritability and anxiety.
- Consider if food allergies or intolerances may be a factor for your child, especially if they are on specialised formulas or you have had to modify your diet (if breastfeeding). The introduction of solids may need to be adapted; seek advice from a child-health nurse or dietitian if you are having any difficulties. *"Food intolerance is a possibility where there is difficulty with any food or you are suspicious of a reaction to any food (in any family member)." Joan Breakey, dietitian.*

- Ensure your child does not eat too close to sleeping periods. A horizontal or semi-horizontal position may affect digestion and trigger reflux.
- Consider offering your child a drink of water after they eat as this may help to wash down any acid from the oesophagus. It may also help dilute any acid in their mouth.
- Feed your child away from other family members (before or after family mealtimes) if they seem too distracted.
- If you are feeling stressed, have your partner, family member or friend feed your child. You may prefer to go for a walk so you do not have to watch.
- Try using music; experiment with which melodies work best (it may soothe you too).
- If you are comfortable with the idea, consider using a dummy during feeds, taking it out and replacing it with a spoon.
- Establish fun eating habits and give lots of encouragement and positive reinforcement to add to the pleasurable experience (e.g. let them play with the food and spoon, give them their own spoon, have a game using the bowl or bib after the feed, or use a bowl with a picture and talk to them about it).

*"We devised lots of interesting bribery for eating, like painting a finger- or toenail for each bite of food, giving stickers or stamps, blowing bubbles, giving high-fives etc." Theresa*

- Use distractions like toys, games, singing or talking while you quickly put the food in. If distractions do not work, then try the opposite and have absolutely no distractions.

- If your child refuses to eat, try again in half an hour when they may be hungrier.
- Try changing the scenery (e.g. go to the park to eat). Meal time may be more successful if they are happier or distracted.
- Be aware that frustration is normal, but try not to get too upset or show anger in front of your child. If you feel frustrated, try strategies such as going outside and screaming loudly or bashing pillows.
- Talk about any feeding issues or frustrations with your partner, family or friends, or contact a support group. If issues are severe or continue to cause difficulties, talk to your doctor.

*"I really try and cook him tasty meals and have never given him commercial baby food . . . and then it [hits me hard] because he spits it all out. It makes me so upset."* Jules

*"Cate has always been a comfort eater . . . She demands food ALL the time. Mostly, she grazes, or nibbles at it . . . Having said that, her need to eat always increases when she is refluxing."* Jody

*"He's really enjoying [solids] but I need to get him when he's hungry enough to be interested but not too hungry so he's upset and out of control."* Jules

*"We've been lucky as Georgie LOVES to eat! By allowing her to take her own interest in solids (not pushing her to eat), and keeping to a very simple diet, she's learned that food's great and our only problem is feeding her enough to keep her happy!"* Theresa

# 7

# Feeding: A Dietitian's Perspective

## Introducing Solids to a Reflux Infant
*By Joan Breakey, Specialist Dietitian*
*Allergy & Food Sensitivity*

> The understanding of fussiness as a developmental pro-
> gression in eating was developed by Joan while working
> with very fussy, food-sensitive infants and children (from
> work beginning in the 1970s), and presented to the
> Reflux Infants Support Association Inc in 1997 with an
> awareness that these issues are even more important in
> infants with reflux.

Parents of infants with reflux can be bombarded with information about how to feed their infant and when and how
to introduce solids. It is of paramount importance to keep in
mind:

- Every reflux infant is different. Just as the position an
  infant is most comfortable being held varies with each
  infant, so there is variation where feeding is concerned.
  The following suggestions will help you think about each
  idea and see how it applies to your infant.

- Any change in anything to do with food is wisest if done GRADUALLY. Do not be surprised if even a very small change in a food means your infant is less comfortable. It does not mean that food is a problem. Read the suggestions below and see what may make the difference for your child.

---

*If an adult with reflux can eat pieces of plain boiled potato but gag if it is mashed, we can appreciate how problematic a small change may be for an infant.*

---

Solids may be introduced if your infant does not seem to be thriving on milk alone or does not seem to be satisfied or settled after feeds, to help with the management of reflux, to see if your infant is food sensitive, and also to very gradually introduce him/her to a range of different foods. Their introduction can be difficult in an infant with reflux because:

- The introduction of solids is not always easy, even for infants without reflux
- There are developmental aspects to eating; just as children vary in speech or coordination development, they vary in acceptance of different aspects of food. Working through this is important for comfort as well as progress
- Reflux can affect all aspects of eating; note in particular the suggestions that relate to thickness, texture, volume and temperature of new foods as they are introduced
- Food sensitivity may be a concern. Read the information on food sensitivities, and be watchful as you progress. This may need to be dealt with, not only if eczema or diarrhoea are present, but because managing food sensitivity will help with the reflux itself.

An infant begins with milk which is bland, smooth, thin, and warm; a normal mixed diet is complex in many aspects. When these aspects are dissected, there are several areas of progression in food acceptance which are developmental. This can help people realise how an infant may be accepting new tastes but not progressing where thicker or scratchier food is concerned. It can help to understand that a child who seems to be 'a difficult eater' or 'very fussy' may just be one who is developing more slowly in one area of eating progression. Parents can look at where the problem is and decide which single area is most relevant, and make gradual changes.

You can decide on the best time to begin solids in your infant, but please speak with your doctor or child-health nurse if you have any concerns. If your infant is thriving, breastmilk or formula can be the complete food for at least nine months, but you may want to begin at six months so you can take your time to advance slowly, or begin earlier if your doctor recommends. Remember that this is an education process where your infant learns to eat, and that is a significant development for any infant. There is no hurry. Increasing variety is not as important as maximising what your child can manage, according to the ideas in this chapter. Milk remains the main source of nutrition for several months.

Your infant is most likely to accept any change when hungry so give solids e.g. rice cereal before a feed, expecting only small amounts to be taken at first. Please note: use rice cereal with no added spice. Later, you may like to introduce a small amount of a new food mixed with a previously accepted food, such as potato with rice cereal, then more of the previously accepted foods (e.g. the rice cereal alone, then the milk feed).

## Some Important Ideas to Help Prevent Fussy Eaters

*By Joan Breakey, Specialist Dietitian*
*Allergy & Food Sensitivity*

> The information below is directed at infants; however, it is still relevant for older age groups.

There are several areas of eating through which each infant has to develop. Understanding these can prevent a lot of frustration and help parents deal with those of most importance to their infant. Some infants seem to sail through eating with no problems at all but others have varying degrees of normal progression.

Reflux infants may be more sensitive to all aspects of feeding than other infants, depending on their level of discomfort and how well treatments are working, so don't worry if they don't progress as quickly. They may have a sensitivity to many aspects, such as tastes and texture change, as well as to sound, light, touch and smell. Maybe others in the family do too. Family sensitivity to any food or smells is an indicator that food sensitivity may be present. Read the article "Is Your Reflux Infant (or Older Child) Food Sensitive?" in this chapter.

Only change ONE aspect of a food at a time. Choose the most important area and work on a small achievable change. Do not expect your child to like food in exactly the same way as you do. Many different forms can be tried, but if this is not accepted then change thickness, temperature, etc. Sometimes children follow family patterns but sometimes they surprise us by being quite different about things.

**1. Taste:** Every new taste is a significant step for a child. We may think rice cereal or potato hasn't much taste but all new tastes are important to an infant. As well as noting acceptance of the new food, also watch for any adverse reaction.

- Add each new taste very gradually to existing bland, accepted food (such as adding mashed potato or rice cereal to milk, if they've only had milk), increasing the amount over seven days.
- Keep food at exactly the same temperature as the accepted milk.
- All infants prefer sweet foods, and recognise the sweetness of cereals and fruit. Use this idea to help introduce new tastes or when you want to encourage them to eat when their reflux is bad.

**2. Texture:** This relates to the feel of the food in the mouth. The major delay in food acceptance is to rough or textured foods, but even bland mashed potatoes or rice cereal have a texture that is difficult for some. If you have found a thickener for milk that helps, use some in solids just while you are making the change to some new food. Expect your reflux infant to progress with changes in texture very slowly. Progressing from smooth/thin to smooth/thick to soft/lumpy to firmer/lumpy can be a long process. Bubbles in soft drink are rejected by some children.

- Change texture very gradually.
- It is important not to change taste and texture together.
- Allow time for your infant to accept smooth potato or rice cereal. Commercial baby food companies put much effort into texture so sometimes infants prefer commercial food. Use them, or use together with homemade

food since the overall plan is that they accept the food the family eats.

**3. Temperature:** Some children are very sensitive to small changes, rejecting mildly warmer or cooler than usual food. Others reject cold food; even sweet, smooth ice-cream.

- Try any new food at milk temperature first. If the meal takes a while it may help to warm the food again.
- Later move gradually to room temperature, then cooler so that your infant can try to handle food from the fridge.
- Each child has their preferred range of accepted temperatures. It takes time to teach well-meaning relations to attend to this too!

**4. Thickness:** Change from milk has to be gradual. If you have thickened milk to help with reflux, use that thickness as your beginning point with solid foods. Many parents know that any change in the thickness of the baby cereal can greatly affect acceptance, but like the above areas, this is still very important when other foods are introduced.

- A not-accepted food may be eaten with only a very small change in thickness.
- Increase thickness while food is still smooth before beginning lumpy food.

**5. Smell:** Sensitive infants and those who are easily nauseated dislike strong smells. As temperature increases, smell increases. If this is a factor for your child, minimise the amount of cooking smells or feed your infant away from the kitchen. As well as strength of smell, consider ingredients such as herbs, spices, onions and garlic. Do not introduce these while there are any problems with food acceptance. Progress may also be affected, or even delayed by, stale, mouldy, aged and 'off' smells; just as new tastes are significant steps, so are new or strong smells.

- An older child may say a food "smells yuk!" but an infant cannot tell us. Reducing the smell by cooling the food may help. Opening a window or using an exhaust fan after cooking can help.
- Use sensitivity to smell in other family members as a guide, or watch your infant's reaction when smells are strong. Reduce smells as much as possible if he/she reacts.

**6. Appearance:** This is probably not important to a very young infant, but becomes important through the pre and primary school years. An infant begins with a narrow range of food and utensils but the child has to progress to a wide variety of presentation forms with different utensils and new situations. Often rejection of foods from other cultures is made on the look of the food. The colour of drinks or food can affect acceptance.

- If a small change in a utensil can upset a child, managing it should be recognised as a developmental leap. You may like to carry your infant's usual bowl and spoon with you if this is a problem.
- Progress does need to occur but your child should be prepared. It is a good idea to proactively make small changes in the colour of the bowl, the utensil, or the place of feeding with no change in the food, so your child can adapt to necessary changes when they have to occur.

**7. Thirst:** Just as it is a progression to add solids to a diet of milk, it is also progression to manage diluted milk and to progress to drinking water. Gradual separation of thirst from hunger is an important step. Over time children need help to clarify that when they are thirsty they need fluid, preferably water, not food. This also aids weight control, since unnecessary food is not eaten.

- If water is not accepted, provide gradually more diluted milk (separate from regular milk feeds) so your infant eventually manages water.

**8. Hunger:** Your infant is much less likely to cope with any new or changed food unless he or she is hungry. It also affects the amount eaten. Attend to any pain or discomfort; hunger will not develop while pain is present. Give small amounts of favoured foods until pain has passed. The amount can be increased after pain is managed.

- Allow time to elapse so that hunger is allowed to develop before expecting your child to manage any change in food. Time elapsed not only relates to recent food, including a rusk, but also to recent drinks such as milk or fruit juice.
- Being able to cope with hunger varies so it is important to very gradually allow your infant to wait while you heat food and bring it to them.

**9. Chewing:** Food to chew on must be provided as gums become firmer from the beginning of teething. Chewing requires effort and will not be attempted if your child is not hungry.

- Use rusks or smooth bones that your infant can hold. Keep attending to this area throughout their first two years, and continue on until your child can manage hard food (e.g. carrot) or fibrous food (e.g. fresh coconut).

**10. The Amount of Food at Meals:** Do not put more food on the plate than you think your child will eat. You may have a teaspoon of the newly changed food, and the accepted amount of the food managed. You will both feel good when it is all gone. The amount should increase as your child grows. They may want less food when in a bad cycle; remember that with less food in their stomach, the less there is to reflux.

- Begin with very small amounts. The remainder can be frozen in iceblock trays and presented next meal or next day.

**11. Time between Meals:** This increases from three hours in infancy to six or more hours in adulthood, with increasing time with no food through the night. The time managed between meals is probably a reflection of metabolic maturity, appreciating that infants have high needs for growth, and little reserves if not fed regularly. It is a big step for an infant to sleep through the night, but take care that small, lean children are not fasting more than twelve hours overnight. There is variation in each individual's ability to fast, depending on needs for growth, activity and inherited metabolic rate. Some do a big catch-up when they wake up.

- At first provide solids before main mealtimes. Gradually move towards usual family mealtimes so you ensure there is food presented at breakfast time, mid-morning, lunch, mid-afternoon and evening meals. Be aware that some parents report reflux is worse one hour after the feed. Note your infant's position after meals, and always prepare everything so you can hold him/her upright longer after feeding.

**12. Other Developmental Progressions:** Remember that just as the rate of speech, motor, emotional and intellectual development varies in different children, so does eating development. Expect your child to progress to the level they are functioning at in other areas (e.g. coordination); if there are other problems, eating will progress more slowly. (Children can be greatly helped by physiotherapy, occupational therapy, and speech therapy. Diet therapy can ensure eating development also progresses.)

- Oral-motor development: affects ability to transfer food from front to back of the mouth, chewing and swallowing. The stage where infants put everything in their mouth may be an important stage in eating development, as they are learning the feel of objects in their mouth. When your infant is young, place food on the back of their tongue to aid swallowing.

- Motor development: may affect posture and ability to transfer finger foods to their mouth. Some infants who have shown no interest in mashed food will surprise you in the way they will take to finger foods. Cope with messiness while development occurs! Watch progress and discuss any delays you notice with your doctor

*"Georgie is . . . stubborn and refused anything to do with food point blank until she was given 'control' of the situation with finger foods." Theresa*

- Emotional development: growth towards independence may be shown by infants wanting to feed themselves or by throwing the food! If your child has a new sibling their overall development may not progress for a time, and eating development may also stall or regress. Each child has a different personality. Some are placid, some do not like change much, and others really enjoy change. Some prefer more of one mixture, and others may prefer some vegetables, some fruit and some cereal.

- If your child is interested in what is on your plate, let them taste some if you think they are ready, or feed them some of their food from your plate.
- Have your child eat with other children so they see others eating and it may encourage them to try new foods.

• Intellectual development: aids understanding of the feeding process, especially understanding that if preparation by a parent or caregiver has begun, food will come soon. Development can happen in stages. Your child may not seem to be accepting new foods for a while then progress may speed up.

- If eating progress and other milestones seem delayed, talk to your doctor.

**13. Learning How to Drink with Meals to Add to Comfort When Eating:** When infants are drinking milk, the proportion of nutrients to fluid is managed, as it is a liquid. When they start solids you can help your infant by giving teaspoons of water, or sips from a cup often throughout the meal so the food is moistened and easier to swallow, and so produces less discomfort.

• Gagging is a primitive reflex to prevent choking. It occurs when the volume of solids in the mouth is too much or when a sensitive infant reacts to a particular texture. It is also an example of individual variation as some people gag very easily with only a small increase in the volume in the mouth or in the thickness of the food.

- Attention to the increase in thickness, lumpiness and volume can reduce gagging. If this does not happen, some children may vomit all the food they have just eaten.
- Progress in a gagging child can be slower in thickness and lumpiness, though new tastes may be accepted well.

**Important Points**
- Aim for a 'good enough diet' first.
- Effort put into nutrition should not be so great that it disrupts family harmony, or spoils the pleasure of family meals. You may prefer to put most effort into giving new foods at lunch, but give accepted food with the family in the evening.
- Call food not accepted 'food your child is not ready for yet', rather than disliked, as this alters the expectation that this cannot change. If the word disliked is used then be specific e.g. scrambled eggs, not eggs generally. A disliked food is one that has been tried in several different forms, thicknesses, temperatures, as described above. Many infants who dislike scrambled eggs (which smell) are quite happy to eat hard boiled eggs (which have little smell).
- If you think your child has an adverse reaction to a food, see your doctor then see a dietitian. You can make a plan to introduce best-tolerated foods first and clarify what foods can be eaten. Children with food allergy may vomit or posset more than if it is just reflux. Adverse reactions to food are easier to manage when your infant is young, rather than putting up with some problems and having to deal with them later, when reactions are worse or involve behavioural symptoms.

People sometimes feel they should manage feeding delay on

their own, but where difficulties occur it is just as appropriate to seek out professional help in this area as it is with other areas of delay. The above ideas show how you can attend to all the issues, and if you have a problem you can decide what to change to improve acceptance. Further help is available if you need it.

## Introduction to Food Sensitivities

Food allergies and intolerances are a factor for many children with reflux. A food allergy involves the body's immune system, which reacts to a food it perceives as harmful; a food intolerance is also a reaction to food, but does not involve the immune system. Food allergies show on allergy tests but there are no tests for food intolerance. Either can cause symptoms of reflux in susceptible children.

If you suspect your child has food sensitivities, talk to your doctor and seek advice from a dietitian. A large number of infants with reflux have cow's milk protein allergy, although other food proteins can sometimes be an issue. Food sensitivity includes both allergy and sensitivity to food additives and other natural chemicals as well.

*"When I tried Alex on a cow's milk-based formula he screamed for four hours." Sharon*

*"Kell can't tolerate dairy or soy protein, which is very different to lactose intolerance . . . [this] limits my diet considerably . . . as I am still breastfeeding . . . Anyway, for the effort I make (huge) I do see results that make it worthwhile. Before we changed his diet he was waking [frequently at] night . . . He wouldn't eat much at all so he was constantly hungry for breast-milk. He would scream and claw at me to be picked up, but once I picked him up, he would lurch around like he wanted to*

*be put down. He would whinge CONSTANTLY and never played independently. He refused food and was just so difficult. It took a month or so to see a good improvement and you've got to be strict, but if it works, it is so worth it." Jules*

*"[Our paediatrician] decided to take Em off all food, feed her elemental formula by naso-gastric tube, let her symptoms settle, then reintroduce foods . . . Within a few days . . . we noticed improvements, and within six weeks she was a new kid. Her vocabulary and comprehension skyrocketed; she was happy, sleeping well and a pleasure to be around." Theresa*

## Is Your Reflux Infant (or Older Child) Food Sensitive?

*By Joan Breakey, Specialist Dietitian Allergy & Food Sensitivity, author of* Are you Food Sensitive?

It is a joy for parents to have a normal healthy infant. Unfortunately not everyone is so lucky. Some parents have to cope with an infant who seems distressed, cries often, and has reflux. With many people talking about allergies and food intolerance, it is not surprising for parents to ask themselves if their infant is food sensitive.

### What Symptoms Can Food-Sensitive Infants Get?

Food may be a factor in diarrhoea, tummy pain, irritability, difficulty settling, poor feeding, sleeplessness and excessive activity as well as in eczema, asthma, sinus and, yes, reflux is a symptom that may also respond to dietary investigation.

### Which Infants Are Most Likely to Be Sensitive?

Those infants most likely to be food sensitive are in families with others who have allergic-type symptoms. These symptoms *do not need to be reactions to specific foods* – it is merely the presence of such symptoms that makes food sensitivity much more likely. If anyone in the family has or had eczema, migraine, irritable bowel syndrome, hayfever, asthma, hives or has a known reaction to a food, the chances are significantly increased that food sensitivity may be a factor.

## When Should I Consider If My Child is Food Sensitive?

Some of these problems are part of the normal ups and downs of infancy. There are very few infants who sleep like angels, and never seem restless or irritable! However, when such symptoms are causing your infant or your family a certain amount of distress, and have been present for some time, then it is worth the effort to find out if there is a solution.

If a problem is significant, the first port of call should be your family doctor. It can be a wonderful relief if you are told that there is no major medical condition present. However, you will still want help in addressing the problem symptom itself. An investigation of food sensitivity may well prove helpful. Alternatively, your infant may suffer from a mild case of several of the above symptoms. There may be some colic and irritability, a little trouble with your infant not settling and not sleeping well, and getting an occasional rash. While you may not feel your infant's discomfort demands medical investigation, you may still wonder if their comfort or sleeping habits may be improved. Ask other parents you know for tips and talk to your child-health nurse. Again, in this case, diet investigation may prove beneficial.

## How Does Food Sensitivity Show?

Sometimes food sensitivity shows clearly. Since infants usually have cow's milk and other foods introduced one at a time, a child who has a clear reaction closely connected to a new whole food can be helped quickly. Alternatively, a child who is given a coloured and flavoured paediatric syrup and reacts badly may also prove easy to assist (though such reactions are sometimes attributed to whatever problem the paediatric syrup was supposed to fix!).

However, sensitivity may be less than obvious because many infants do not react until several days after the problem food has been introduced, or when there is a build-up to a certain threshold from different problem foods. In these cases, food sensitivity can be detected through a process of elimination and subsequent reintroduction of many suspect foods.

## What Can Be Done If I Decide Food Sensitivity May Be Present?

Once the presence of food sensitivity seems possible, it is wise to keep a written record of symptoms and foods introduced, with your infant's age. It becomes difficult to remember events later, especially as progress is often complicated by other happenings in the family. This information on changes in food and symptoms provide leads in 'diet detective work', so professionals can begin to clarify what substances to check on, and you'll feel more secure in your quest to investigate food sensitivity.

Your doctor may suggest a dietitian who will help you design an initial 'family detective diet' of minimally suspect foods, to see if diet is involved in your infant's problems. If you feel confident working on your own, a book such as *Are You Food Sensitive?* (which outlines the process in a detailed, step-by-step fashion, and has sections referring specifically to food sensitivity in infants) may be helpful. You will find the detective work will get broader as you learn to watch out not only for foods, but for smells, flavoured or coloured medications or vitamins, and other factors.

Sometimes well-meaning relations, friends and professionals imply that you shouldn't consider food sensitivity, as they think it is just an idea that is fashionable but without substance. This is not true! If you think your child may be food sensitive, please persist. If you know someone who would like to investigate diet in their child, please support them.

## Diet Therapy

The family detective diet: Diet therapy is not just having general information on a sheet of paper. You need professional help in the confusing area of replacing one food with another, and in planning exactly what to eat in the elimination diet, especially as food-sensitive infants are individuals and can be very fussy eaters. Sometimes it is necessary to completely exclude foods, but fortunately the intake of some foods may just need decreasing. Small amounts of these decreased foods, with the freely allowed foods, can give sufficient variety. Once your infant has been on the family detective diet for four weeks, and the symptoms have decreased, diet therapy emphasises gradual reintroduction of low-risk foods over the oncoming months. As important as the initial step of finding out that your infant is food sensitive, reintroduction of low-risk foods is equally significant, as carefully controlled and monitored reintroduction of foods can ensure that your infant is on the least strict diet possible. In this way, the family can be sure that they are not going to a lot of effort to totally exclude a food, when it might be managed in small doses, or when it is cooked a certain way. If the elimination diet does not appear to have made any difference, reintroduce all excluded foods and additives for seven full days to clarify if diet has no role. Sometimes bad days come back and more investigation can be done.

The 'total body load': The addition of additives and suspect whole foods to environmental factors creates a 'total body load'. When all are reduced sufficiently to decrease symptoms they can gradually be reintroduced. The diet may need to be used more strictly in spring when coping with pollen, or when teething or infections are present. On the bright side, the diet can be relaxed when such factors are not present.

Smells that may be problematic include all perfumes such as those in laundry items, air fresheners, and perfumed insect repellents, as well as paint, varnish or petrol, in fact, anything which smells, even natural flowers and herbs.

Medications for infants are usually given as syrups which are usually coloured and flavoured. Of course the illness producing the need for the medication can make your infant irritable, but it is important to report any additional changes to your doctor after medication is begun. Also note in your 'detective book' whether changes coincided with overtiredness, changes in weather, or stress in the family. One way to look at food sensitivity is to consider that food may be an aggravating factor in the child's environment. If stress is present, the food sensitivity symptoms will be worse, so maximum improvement occurs when both diet and family stress are addressed.

The diet changes over time: Food sensitivity does change over time, especially in the first years of a child's life. The good news is that tolerance usually increases with age! It is good to see two to three year olds tolerating carefully controlled amounts of food that produced adverse symptoms in infancy. On the other hand, sometimes the problem food can remain the same, but the type of symptom aggravated can change. Many parents who seek assistance with diet investigation when there are concentration problems in a school-age child, having put up with behavioural problems in preschool, earaches as a toddler, and reflux or colic in infancy say they wish they had known so they could have begun diet investigation several years earlier.

Remember that: in food-sensitive people, diet aggravates the underlying tendency. If diet investigations are begun in infancy when reactions are clearer, the family can learn what foods the child manages. Too many families are told their infant 'will grow out of it' when diet would have greatly decreased the initial problem, not just the similar or additional problems that have arisen in later years.

### What If My Infant is Not Getting Enough to Eat?

A natural concern of most parents when beginning investigation for food sensitivity is ensuring that their infant is still well fed. In the effort to find out what is causing a problem it is easy to look mostly at what should be excluded and not notice sufficiently what is left in. Sometimes families become more and more worried about foods until there are very few left. If this occurs, we then have the problem of your infant being even more distressed because of hunger. With professional help this need never occur, as there are always alternative foods to be found, and small amounts of problem foods are often tolerated with specific cooking methods.

### Milk

Since milk is so important, especially in the first six months of an infant's life, it deserves special consideration. Milk should always be considered as suspect if at any time your infant or a close relative has, or previously had, a reaction to it. It is also important to consider what solids may have been introduced into your infant's diet so that milk is not blamed for the symptoms when they may be due to some other food.

Breastfeed if possible: Just as we know that breastfed infants benefit from the variety of flavours that come through breast-milk, food-sensitive infants can have adverse reactions to those flavours and other chemicals. Allergens also come through breastmilk and although no infant is allergic to the protein in their mother's milk they could react to something in the milk. It is important to realise that a mother does not need to give up breastfeeding if her infant is distressed in some way. The solution is for Mum to go on an elimination diet suited to her. It is very important that professional help is used to ensure that Mum is eating well enough for her own needs, as well as for adequate milk production. All infants, especially distressed ones, are most helped by a caring mother who takes the time to look after herself and ensure she is not getting rundown. Foods eaten can be gradually expanded, first by Mum having advice about how she can trial foods via breastmilk, and later by a planned introduction of solids for the infant.

## Allergy to Cow's Milk

If you suspect your infant is sensitive to cow's milk, discuss your concerns with professionals before making any changes. Remember a mother generally does not need to give up breast-feeding, although she may need to exclude all dairy products from her diet. It is important that professional help is used. Any cow's milk formula must be replaced with another suitable infant formula. Sometimes a change from one formula to another helps.

Lactose intolerance is a reaction to the milk sugar. This is different to a milk-protein sensitivity. If lactose intolerance is suspected, discuss this with your doctor. Note that lactose intolerance only produces gut symptoms.

Soy milk formulas are equivalent nutritionally to cow's milk formulas but doctors now recommend they not be used until after six months of age. A change to soy solves the problem for many infants, though about half of those allergic to dairy are also allergic to soy. Discuss how to test it with your dietitian so that very gradual introduction is managed.

Goat's milk formulas are sometimes trialled by families, though goat's milk protein is similar to cow's milk protein, and the adverse symptoms that occurred with cow's milk often re-appear around six weeks after use is begun. On the other hand, if goat's milk formula is tolerated, then cow's milk can later be gradually reintroduced.

Partially hydrolysed formulas (Nan HA, S26 HA) are infant milk formulas where the protein is partially broken down (hydrolysed). These formulas may be useful where there is a risk of allergies or where the symptoms are not very troublesome. Where a dairy allergy is suspected, or where the allergy is mild, these formulas may still be useful, but use only on the advice of your doctor and/or dietitian.

> *"Milk tolerance varies depending on how much the protein is changed. As a dietitian, I have met people on farms who have reported reactions to fresh milk but not to pasteurised milk, others who cannot tolerate pasteurised but manage UHT milk, yet others who cannot tolerate milk unless it is cooked (e.g. evaporated milk or cappuccino coffee), some who can only manage a HA formula, some who can only tolerate the extensively hydrolysed formulas, and those more allergic who can tolerate only amino acid-based formulas."*
> *Joan Breakey*

## Allergy to Cow's Milk and Soy

Where infants are allergic to both dairy and soy, do not despair! The formulas listed below are available on a doctor's prescription (they are very expensive without one). It is important to work with professionals as your infant needs to be under the care of a doctor and dietitian to manage the diet detective work of managing food trials and nutrition.

Extensively hydrolysed formulas (Alfaré, Pepti-Junior) are infant-milk formulas where the protein is more fully broken down (further hydrolysed).

Amino acid-based formulas (EleCare, Neocate) are elemental formulas where the protein is completely hydrolysed into its most broken-down form. Almost all children tolerate them, but because they taste quite bitter the change from the previously used formula should be very gradual, over seven to fourteen days. Some infants drink them anyway as the adverse symptoms are relieved. The bitterness may be able to be disguised initially by using sugar or golden syrup, if necessary. Vanilla is sometimes suggested, but is not recommended because some infants are sensitive to it.

## Vitamins and Minerals

Some people ask about the role of vitamins and minerals in food sensitivity. These nutrients can be supplied in a normal diet. Food sensitivity is not due to a deficiency of nutrients, so adding them in is not a solution. In fact, it can become another confusing factor in the detective work of things which could be affecting your infant, especially as most vitamins and minerals are flavoured.

## The Solution

When food sensitivity exists, a change in the diet can seem like magic. But it is rarely an easy treatment. It takes time and effort to keep going over a long time, and it is not easy to cope with food being offered by well-intentioned relations and friends. However, as long as the problem symptoms are minimised, parents report that their infant's increased comfort more than balances the additional effort. Sometimes parents forget how bad the situation used to be and relax the diet. It can be quite therapeutic for them to suddenly be reminded!

## Summary

The general recommendations with regard to food sensitivity are listed below:

- Do not exclude any food from a child's diet without good reason, preferably clarifying this with professional help.
- When you have had help planning an elimination diet, take care to exclude all of the suspect foods for a full four-week period so you have a good diet baseline from which to start trialling new foods.
- Remember that diet detective work also includes the environment. Attention to the 'total body load' may show when the diet needs to be more strictly adhered to and when it can be relaxed.
- You are unlucky if the exclusions have to be forever! Most infants improve in their tolerance. Seek professional help for continual new ideas and gradual broadening of the diet. Carefully managed reintroduction of low suspect foods can occur over time as challenges, so the diet can be as practical and easy as possible.
- Obtain allergy testing if possible and be guided by your allergist about action. If the allergy is severe then complete avoidance is necessary. Retesting over years may show decreased reactivity.

- Foods are not always eliminated completely, or allowed in an unlimited way. The dietitian can often help you so that some foods are able to be tolerated in small amounts if cooked in a particular way, depending on your child's level of tolerance and the total body load of suspect items.
- Non-severe reactions still need attention. A dietitian can advise how to gradually trial foods using methods that mean food tolerance is maximised.

## Older Children

Investigating possible food sensitivities in older children follows the same ideas. Those most likely to respond to dietary investigation for food sensitivity include those who have any or all of the following: an allergic family history as mentioned above, as well as having some of another group of symptoms (headaches, tummy aches, mouth ulcers, car sickness, limb pains, sleep problems, nightmares, mood changes, attention-deficit hyperactivity disorder or autistic spectrum disorder); a family member who has an adverse reaction to aspirin, an increased sensitivity to smell (both in food and in the environment), an increased sensitivity to taste; and those who have seen a definite adverse reaction to a food or additive in the past. They may have increased body odour or bad breath. Food sensitivity is not related to any particular diagnosis. It relates to whether members of that family have reactions or not. See the book *Are You Food Sensitive?* for more information.

There is still much that is unknown about food sensitivity. The problems may be solved easily, or you may benefit from professional help. If you suspect that your child is food sensitive, talk to your child-health nurse or doctor, and ring a dietitian. Some dietitians specialise in this area of diet therapy, so you can solve the problems faster. It is so good when symptoms improve!

Are You Food Sensitive? *by Joan Breakey is available through RISA Inc or via Joan Breakey's website at www.ozemail. com.au/~breakey.*

> *"Many mums have had success breastfeeding and doing an elimination diet . . . They can really make a difference for baby. Sometimes mums even find out they feel much better if they eliminate certain foods (I'm one of those)."*

> *"The biggest discovery (besides sorting out their food allergies) was to learn about Multiple Chemical Sensitivity and realising that our two little girls suffered from it – a simple shopping trip can result in a major reaction that can include reflux as a symptom. Thankfully, getting the allergies and chemical sensitivity under control has seen the end of our reflux days." Theresa*

# 8

# Feeding: A Speech Pathologist's Perspective

## Concerns Regarding Infant Feeding Patterns

*By Dr Julie Cichero, deglutitionist (feeding and swallowing therapist) and speech pathologist.*

Parents know their children better than anyone. If you have concerns regarding your child's feeding habits or feeding milestones, please speak with your doctor. Your local doctor or child-health nurse can provide information regarding expected growth and weight-gain patterns. Please note: the following symptoms should be brought to your doctor's attention:

- increased breathing effort during or after eating
- increased breathing rate after feeding (fast, short breaths)
- wet 'gurgly' voice during or after eating
- colour changes around their mouth/face (e.g. pale or blue)
- unexplained chest infections
- reflux/vomiting during or after eating
- poor weight gain.

Your doctor will be able to advise you of any measures that may be required. They may refer your child to other medical specialists for further investigations, or to other health professionals, such as a speech pathologist or dietitian if required. In addition, you are encouraged to speak with a health professional if your child displays any of the symptoms below:

- regularly taking longer than thirty minutes to complete feeds
- difficulty sucking during breast or bottle feeds
- irritability or sleepiness during feeding
- gagging or choking on solid foods
- food refusal.

## Health Professionals with Experience in Infant Feeding Issues

> This list is not exhaustive. Your doctor can provide you with referrals to other health professionals as necessary. The health professionals listed below may also provide other services; and those in the private sector generally do not require a letter of referral.

**1. Speech pathologists** are able to provide advice regarding:

- breast or bottle feeding issues
- suck – swallow – breathing co-ordination for breast and bottle fed infants
- lips, tongue and jaw positioning for breastfed infants, including assistance with attachment
- assistance with pacing
- (for bottle fed infants) the most appropriate teat and bottle to suit your infant

- transitional feeding problems (delay in starting solids, difficulty managing lumpy foods, etc)
- behavioural feeding problems related to illness
- oral stimulation and oral de-sensitisation for infants who have had unpleasant bodily experiences (e.g. vomiting) and invasive nasal tubes, and to assist with later transitions to food by mouth
- assistance with programmes to acquire chewing skills, if developmental chewing skills are delayed or absent (unsafe chewing practices can exacerbate gagging and choking).

Not all speech pathologists provide services for infants with feeding problems. You will need to clarify this when you arrange an appointment. Public services are available at children's hospitals or attached to disability services units. Private speech pathologists are listed in the telephone book or with Speech Pathology Australia at www.speechpathologyaustralia.org.au.

**2. Dietitians** are able to provide advice regarding:
- volume of feed intake required to meet calorie and nutrient requirements
- (for bottle-fed infants) the most appropriate formula to suit your infant
- diet changes necessary in response to food allergies or intolerances
- nutritional advice for breastfeeding mothers to ensure optimum breastmilk production
- ideas on food texture and other factors that affect reflux

Not all dietitians provide services for infants with feeding problems. You will need to clarify this when you arrange an appointment. Public services are available at major public hospitals. Private Accredited Practicing Dietitians can be contacted via the Dietitians Association of Australia at www.daa.asn.au or by phone on 1800 812 942.

**3. Lactation Consultants** promote and assist with breastfeeding. They offer support and specialist assistance to mothers who wish to breastfeed. They are able to provide advice regarding:

- establishing and maintaining breastmilk supply (in the best interests of mother and child/children)
- attachment at the breast
- breastfeeding difficulties experienced by infants and toddlers.

Public services may be available at major public hospitals. Private lactation consultants are listed in the telephone book or with Australian Lactation Consultants Association of Australia Inc at www.alca.asn.au. As an ongoing support network, the Australian Breastfeeding Association at www.breastfeeding.asn.au may also be able to assist.

**4. Child Health Nurses** are able to provide services that include:

- health-care assessment, health information and education
- parent education and guidance in relation to breastfeeding and/or general feeding and nutrition issues, normal growth and developmental milestones, speech development, oral health, immunisation, safety issues, coping with sleep and settling and routines
- assessment of emotional and physical wellbeing of the family
- early intervention and/or referral to the appropriate service providers

- families with links within their community and to other services such as community parenting groups.

Community health centres are located throughout Australia. Your local doctor should be able to provide information regarding your closest centre.

**5. Residential Services** (e.g. Ellen Barron Family Centre; Tresillian Family Care Centres) may offer day-stay and week-stay programs for parents and their infants. This service assists parents who require more intensive support with parenting issues that include:

- coping with the new role of mum or dad
- establishing routines
- establishing and/or maintaining breastfeeding
- feeding issues including the introduction of solids or managing fussy eaters, sleeping and settling issues, and toddler behavioural issues
- coping with depression and anxiety, relationship issues.

Your doctor/child nurse can advise whether you would benefit from attending services at these centres, and will organise a referral if necessary.

## GOR and Feeding Development

*By Dr Julie Cichero, deglutitionist (feeding and swallowing therapist) and speech pathologist*

Some children have difficult behaviours during feeding or they may present with delayed feeding skills. Assistance can be provided by speech pathologists who specialise in paediatric feeding and swallowing problems (not all speech pathologists or dietitians work in this specialised area).

## What Kinds of Developmental Feeding Problems or Behaviours do Children with Gastro-Oesophageal Reflux Show?

### 1. Breast or Bottle feeding

Infants may demonstrate:

- an inability to take more than a small volume of feed (e.g. fifty to seventy millilitres per feed). This is despite showing clear hunger cues and an eagerness to feed, but then rejection of the breast or bottle after a short time and small volume
- increasing irritability/fussing throughout the feed. Infants may demonstrate struggling behaviours such as back-arching, crying, pushing back, head-turning, pulling off the bottle or breast and refusing attempts to re-attach
- crying/screaming soon after commencing the feed or struggling when they are put into a feeding position (either breast/bottle)
- a 'gurgly tummy' during feeds
- consistent effortless vomiting after feeds or projectile vomiting. Vomiting associated with GOR is more likely to occur with your infant lying flat than upright. Note: Vomiting is different to posseting. Posseting is a mixture of milk feed and saliva that may come out of your infant's mouth with a burp or a hiccup. Vomiting shows a larger volume than posseting.

Be aware that even when your infant vomits, even though it looks a lot it is unlikely that the entire feed has been brought up. To test this for yourself, take forty millilitres water and spill it onto the table to get an idea of what it looks and feels like when cleaning up.

## 2. Commencing 'First Solids' (Blended/Pureed Foods)

It is often said that introduction of solids can help to settle a reflux infant because the heavier food is more inclined to stay in the stomach. Talk to your doctor or child-health nurse about the best time to introduce solids to your infant. Whilst the general recommendation is six months of age, some paediatricians recommend starting solids at four months of age. Four months is the earliest an infant should start solids as they do not have the oral motor or breathing and swallowing coordination skills to safely manage solids prior to this age. Some infants who have experienced reflux may also experience difficulty commencing first solids. It is important to note that first solids should be quite runny (e.g. like pouring-cream consistency). Your child may have more difficulty with sticky, thick and paste-like purees. These thicker textures require more tongue movement, are heavy in the mouth and may encourage gagging behaviour.

It is normal for an infant to push food out of their mouth the first few days of solids or when new foods are tried. It is normal for infants to make faces when they try first solids. First solids are for practising oral movements. Anticipate that on day one you may only get one teaspoon in; this is fine. Gradually increase the amount of solids offered, being careful to watch for infant cues of when they have had enough. They have little tummies, and too much food will make them feel uncomfortable. Remember that milk (breastmilk or formula) remains essential for the first twelve months.

Some reflux infants may experience discomfort and show behaviours including gagging, vomiting, spitting out; and refusal behaviours (head turning, pushing or throwing food away, clamping shut their mouth, crying or saying "no"). Refusing, head-turning and pushing food away may also be seen when your infant has had some solids and is trying to communicate that they have had enough.

## 3. Commencing 'Lumpy Mashed/Semisolid' Textures

When infants start pureed solids at about four to six months of age, they are generally ready to manage soft lumps at about eight months of age. Some children may have difficulty with this texture and may avoid it altogether due to increased sensitivity (hypersensitivity) in the mouth. These infants may skip lumpy solids and move to chewing on soft solids and safe finger foods. Behaviours may include gagging, vomiting, spitting out; and refusal behaviours (head turning, pushing or throwing food away, clamping shut their mouth, crying or saying "no"). Some children need assistance learning to chew. When a child attempts to swallow whole foods that need chewing, the body's response is to gag to protect the airway from a possible choking risk. Lumpy solids should be placed onto the gums at the side of the mouth to help them learn that this is where lumps need to go. An up-down rudimentary chewing action may be seen.

## 4. Commencing Chewable Foods

Children may start to try dry chewable foods (e.g. shortbread-style biscuits or Cruskits) even though they will completely refuse lumpy semi-solid textures. Early chewing patterns in children with GORD include:

- nibbling tiny amounts of the biscuit, but gagging or vomiting on larger lumps
- mouthing the rusk/fruit stick, etc, then spitting the lumps out of their mouth
- mouthing or trying to 'suck' the material
- tongue-mashing the food in the midline of the mouth

(like a suck pattern) and then gagging or vomiting as it goes over the back of their mouth

- trouble moving the food to the gums on the sides of the mouth so that it can be chewed with molar teeth
- lack of development of mature chewing (e.g. may munch the material in an up-down chewing pattern, but not use a more adult-style rotary chewing movement that shows diagonal jaw movements).

Some children require assistance to learn how to chew. Sucking on food and nibbling tiny amounts indicates that they have not yet learned the skills associated with early chewing. Large lumps will be a cause for gagging. As described above, this is a safety mechanism to prevent choking. Gagging is unpleasant and if parents are upset by the gagging, the child may become upset and frightened. These children need assistance to learn to chew so they feel safe when eating. A paediatric speech pathologist with infant feeding skills can assist with a short program to help children learn to chew.

## How Does GOR Affect Other Types of Development in Children?

Gastro-oesophageal reflux also can affect children's enjoyment and milestones for movement and touch or sensation.

**Movement:** Some infants do not enjoy prone lying (i.e. tummy time); however, some infants with reflux find comfort in this position. Some infants do not like to be moved around, bounced on laps or put into different positions. Infants who are sensitive in this regard may become irritable or even vomit.

**Sensation:** As noted above, frequent vomiting may affect a child's enjoyment and willingness to try lumpy solids or other textured food. Due to discomfort associated with vomiting and also cleaning up, children may become upset or irritable with other forms of sensation. Some will become distressed if their hands are covered in wet or grainy foods or other textures (dry textures are most comfortable for them). These children may pick things up very well with their fingers and thumbs (pincer grip), but dislike touching things across the palms of their hands. They may not hold spoons to feed themselves. They may also dislike the feeling of different textures on their feet and may cry or get distressed when they walk on different surfaces such as grass or sand. Sometimes this heightened sensitivity to touch can extend to discomfort with clothing tags, and dislike of tooth brushing or having hair or nails cut.

**Tube-feeding:** For very severe feeding problems, where there is concern that the infant may not be able to consume enough food/fluid to meet their dietary requirements, children may commence tube-feeding. See the chapter on tube-feeding for further information.

## Everyday Feeding related Activities for Children

*By Dr Julie Cichero, deglutitionist (feeding and swallowing therapist) and speech pathologist*

There are a number of activities that you can engage in every day to assist your child to learn about how we eat food. You may be well aware that infants will crawl, stand, walk with assistance around furniture, and then attempt their own independent first steps. However, you may not be as keenly aware of the steps associated with learning to eat food and food of different tastes and textures.

**1. Eat with your child.** Talk to them about the food and what it is called. Use exaggerated motions to smell the food and describe the smell and taste. Smile and comment on how nice it tastes. Show them exaggerated chewing actions so they can see what you are doing with the food once it is in your mouth.

**2. Encourage children to touch food with their hands.** This can happen at the grocery store when you are choosing fruit and vegetables or when you are preparing food for the evening meal. Give children the words to describe the different touch sensations (e.g. soft, hard, grainy, bumpy, warm, cold, rough, squooshy) and encourage them to say the words with you. Being able to touch different foods with their fingers helps give their brain some prior warning as to what the food might be like in a more sensitive area (e.g. on their lips and then in their mouth).

**3. Encourage imaginative play activities around food.** Encourage children to pretend to feed dolls, puppets and teddies. Children's tea parties provide a wonderful opportunity to pretend with eating, and holding utensils. Some children pretend drinking at bath-time due to the natural abundance of water! These activities give your child a chance to learn skills associated with eating and drinking without the pressure to actually eat or drink anything. As it is non-threatening, they are more likely to want to participate.

**4. Tooth-brushing is an important part of the 'eating ritual'.** First toothbrushes have handles and knobbly rubber ends on them. Children love to chew on the rubber end as it often squeaks. This chewing action provides good exercise for the developing jaw muscles that are needed for managing chewable foods. The knobbly bits also encourage the inquisitive tongue to move around the mouth and to learn that lumps belong on the gums. This is the very first step to learning to chew efficiently. The dexterity of the tongue is as important for feeding as it is for learning to talk. Exercises that improve tongue function work on improving both feeding and early communication skills. Second and third toothbrushes become less rubbery and more like the adult toothbrushes we are familiar with. Tooth-brushing habits started early will stand children in good stead to look after their teeth for life. Teeth are like little knives (biting) and plates used to break the food down. We wash our dishes after meals to have clean plates for the next meal; it makes good sense to brush our teeth twice daily too. Teeth that are cleaned regularly are less likely to develop 'sores' (i.e. cavities/holes). Tooth pain can make eating uncomfortable too.

**5. Take the opportunity to read books and sing songs about food and eating.** Books like *The Very Hungry Caterpillar* and *I Will Never Not Ever Eat a Tomato* in the Clarice Bean series are popular favourites with children and adults.

## Speech Pathology Questions and Answers

*By Dr Julie Cichero, deglutitionist (feeding and swallowing therapist) and speech pathologist*

**1. Question:** "How do you get a stubborn baby girl to accept solids – she just shuts her mouth when she sees any food coming!" Tania

**Answer:** How old is this little one? If she is young (six months) she may not be ready yet. If she is older than six to seven months it is worth having this issue investigated because there is a critical period for development of feeding skills. She may also have oral hypersensitivity, be at risk of things 'going down the wrong way', have food allergies or a range of other problems.

We would encourage lots of mouthing (toys in mouth; fingers in mouth; toothbrush – not necessarily to clean teeth, just acceptance in the mouth; solids like rusk sticks). Sometimes little ones exert their independent personalities very early in life. She may do better with food that she can hold and put in her own mouth. Also, she may already be full (milk) when you offer her the solids. Try offering the solids first and then the milk after (ensure she is hungry).

**2. Question:** "My son will only eat purees as he gags and sometimes vomits on anything else. Is this normal for children with reflux? How long does this last, and how do I encourage new textures?"

**Answer:** This little one may be presenting with a heightened awareness of things going into the mouth (hypersensitivity), which is quite common in little ones with reflux. We would encourage lots of mouthing (see examples in previous answer). As well, toothbrush trainers (available in Woolworths, Coles, and all pharmacies) have textured ends on them that your child can practice biting on.

When introducing solids, the texture needs to be increased very slowly. Use the same food (i.e. keep flavour the same), but gradually make the food thicker (i.e. less water, add rice cereal/corn flour) then lumpier.

To start introducing lumps into purees you could grate a little bit of cheese into the puree, or crumble very small pieces of arrowroot biscuit or day-old bread into the puree. Start with a couple of spoonfuls of smooth puree. Then give them a spoonful of puree with one or two of the little lumps in it, then go back to smooth puree. Gradually increase the number of spoonfuls that have the little lumps in it (over a period of days). You could also sprinkle the rice cereal in (in small amounts) as it also would provide some fine texture and has the benefit of being iron fortified. Try this at a meal early in the day or at lunchtime, rather than dinnertime when you and your child are probably both tired.

If your child gags, remain calm and remove the food. If you react with fright and horror at a small gag, your child learns that this is fearful situation and is thus more likely to gag. Some children do better to avoid this texture and move straight onto finger foods when they are a bit older. If you would like more advice or you are concerned the gagging is very often or poses a choking risk, please seek further detailed assessment by a feeding and swallowing clinician or discuss your concerns with your GP or paediatrician.

## Other Developmental Issues

Children with reflux can sometimes have delays in areas other than feeding and swallowing. If you are concerned that your child is not achieving new skills at the same rate as other children, talk to your doctor or child-health nurse. Your child may benefit from early childhood intervention, which, depending on their needs, may include services such as physiotherapy, occupational therapy, music therapy, audiology and psychology (as well as diet therapy and speech pathology). The sooner the intervention, the better your child's progress is likely to be.

*"We got [Kell's] 'report card' [from daycare]. As expected he did very badly in speech and language and in feeding himself, dressing himself and quite a number of other milestones (walking down stairs, running, recognising colours, etc). I know that with him being so sick [and in pain from reflux] for such a long time means he's got catching up to do so I'm okay with all that. He*

*did quite well in puzzles and in shape-sorting so it's not all bad." Jules*

*"It seems obvious (sensory issues and reflux) are related in many cases. [My son] has been assessed by an Occupational Therapist as his sensory issues have been so bad that changing nappies/ giving a bath, etc, are almost impossible when he is unwell. He bites and can be very aggressive, chokes on food and has language delays, etc. These issues combined can point to a picture of Autistic Spectrum disorder or at least Sensory Integration Disorder. [Our paediatrician] read the OT report and said he thought it was more likely to be reflux-related and that if we resolve those issues, then the sensory and behavioural issues can be addressed and will probably resolve . . . During [periods of wellness] he was able to enjoy being bathed, could walk on textured surfaces, started talking at a staggering rate and stopped biting almost completely. As soon as he gets sick he reverts and life gets very difficult for the family."*

*Acknowledgements to Dr Pamela Dodrill (BSpPath (Hons), PhD) and Ms Kelly Weir (BSpThy, MSpPath), speech pathologists, for their contributions to RISA Inc newsletters. Elements of these contributions have been incorporated into this chapter and are gratefully acknowledged.*

# 9

# Reflux Medication

Use of specific brand names is done to help with the understanding and recognition of different types of medications and is not an endorsement of these drugs. Choice of medication or other treatment should only be a matter for discussion between you and your child's doctor. For pharmaceutical information, contact a pharmacist at your local hospital or pharmacy, or call Medicines Line on 1300 888 763. Further information and resources are available from the National Prescribing Service Ltd at www.nps.org.au.

## Use of Medication

Some infants and children with reflux have symptoms severe enough to warrant treatment beyond simple lifestyle changes. Medication may be the best way of relieving their pain or helping to alleviate their reflux, although not all infants and children will need them.

The choice to use medications may or may not seem obvious. You may wonder what the consequences of medicating your child may be, and what the side effects or long-term effects could be. These are very legitimate concerns, and ones that need to be directed towards your child's doctor or a pharmacist. Also legitimate and equally important to know, are the short and long term consequences of NOT medicating your child and whether this will be a safer option. Even though it may be daunting, medication is something you may need to consider. Please discuss this with your child's doctor if you have any concerns.

> *"Medication was the only thing that gave him any relief and it took a while to get him medicated properly. I think for me I was just so exhausted and there is only so many times you can watch your baby in so much pain before you say give him something. I have been told that leaving severe reflux unmedicated can lead to permanent damage . . . so I guess it's which evil is the lesser? For me also it was a choice of quality of life for him and myself too."*

There are several different types of medications that may be recommended. Generally reflux medications are used to reduce the amount of acid that the oesophagus or respiratory tract is exposed to, to prevent symptoms and promote healing. They may be available over the counter or by prescription. If you are considering giving any over-the-counter medication to your child such as antacids, please seek medical guidance. It is also worth remembering that mixing medications can be dangerous (this includes over-the-counter medications and herbal remedies), so you need to let your doctor and pharmacist know all of the medication your child is taking, whether prescribed or not.

The doctor will take your child's age and the severity of their reflux into consideration when choosing which medications to use. The dosage and combination they judge is right for your child will be based on their experience and preference. Even so, there may be some trial and error involved to find which drugs, alone or in combination, are most suitable. For the best results, most medicines need to be given on a regular basis.

The effects of these medications will be different for each child, with some responding almost immediately whilst others may take several weeks (it may also take longer if there is any irritation or inflammation in the gut). If the medication benefits your child, it should be continued as prescribed by your doctor. The need for continued use of the medication should be periodically reviewed. Even if it does not appear to be having any benefit, continue administering the medication as prescribed and talk to your child's doctor. Lack of response to medication does not indicate that reflux is not the issue. It may simply mean that not enough time has elapsed, or perhaps that medication at that dose may not be right for your child. Discuss any concerns with your doctor or pharmacist.

Medications should be reviewed by your doctor on a regular basis. Some medication dosages are determined by your child's weight and the dose may need to be adjusted as they grow.

---

Your local pharmacist or a compounding pharmacy may be able to provide medication so it can be delivered in a different way such as suspension, and may be able to alter the flavour if its taste is a problem.

---

## Reflux Medications

### Antacids

Antacids (Mylanta Original®, Gastrogel®, Andrews Tums® antacid) offer short-term relief of intermittent symptoms of reflux in children. Most antacids use a combination of different mineral salts to neutralise some of the acid lying free in the stomach. They begin to work quickly, but the effect generally only lasts for a couple of hours.

- Antacids can affect the absorption of other medications. If possible, do not give with other medications. Always seek the advice of the pharmacist or doctor if your child is on antacids and is taking other medication.

- The maximum dose to be given per day should be discussed with your doctor. Medically unsupervised long-term or excessive use can lead to complications.

- Mylanta® Original Formulation is suitable for use in children from one month of age. Other formulations of Mylanta may not be suitable, particularly if your child is taking other reflux medication. Ask your pharmacist or doctor for the correct dose.

## Alginates/Thickening Agents

Alginates/Thickening Agents (Infant Gaviscon®) reduce regurgitation in infants. Infant Gaviscon® thickens the contents of the stomach and makes it more difficult to reflux into the oesophagus.

- Infant Gaviscon® should not be used with other thickening agents or thickened formulas as it can make the stomach contents too thick.

- Liquid Gaviscon® (adult preparation) works differently; it is an antacid which reacts with stomach acid and produces a frothy layer on top of the stomach contents. It is not usually recommended in infants due to its high sodium content.

## Histamine-2 Receptor Antagonists (H2RA or H2 Blockers)

Histamine-2 Receptor Antagonists (ranitidine, Zantac®; cimetidine, Tagamet®), suppress acid production. H2RAs block the action of histamine in the stomach, as histamine stimulates the production and release of acid by specific cells in the stomach wall. This prevents the acid-secreting cells in the stomach from becoming active.

- H2RAs are generally more effective than antacids, but not as effective as Proton Pump Inhibitors (PPIs).
- To be most effective, the dose may need to be reviewed as your child puts on weight.
- If your child will not accept the taste of Zantac® Syrup, ask your doctor if the effervescent tablet is an option. Alternatively, the flavour may be changed by a compounding pharmacist – speak with them for further information.

*"With Zantac, I always do it in a syringe and try and put it into the back of their mouth, near the cheek, as this bypasses a lot of the tastebuds. This way, too, it is over with really quickly."*
*Karen*

## Proton Pump Inhibitors (PPIs)

Proton Pump Inhibitors (omeprazole Losec®; lansoprazole, Zoton®; esomeprazole; Nexium®) enter the acid-secretory cells of the stomach wall (parietal cells) and inhibit the acid-making enzyme in the cell. Put simply, this process stops acid production.

- PPIs are more potent acid suppressants and longer acting than H2RAs.

- For many PPIs, the protective enteric coating is on the granules within the tablets or capsules. It is important the granules are not chewed or crushed as they may become less effective.
- If dispersing PPI granules, make sure you use the correct liquid or puree as directed for the specific PPI. Using the wrong substance may alter its effectiveness.
- If your child vomits with their reflux, PPIs will not change that. PPIs suppress acid production in the stomach so that any vomiting will not hurt as much.

*"We dissolved Losec in a small amount of water, either in a small container or on a Zantac medicine spoon . . . My son's been taking Losec like this since he was six weeks old." Karen*

*"I put the Losec into a Nurofen syringe (the hole is larger than other syringes) and suck up some cooled boiled water." Michelle*

*"When we changed the time Ewan took his Nexium, we saw a lot of difference." Janine*

## Prokinetic Agents (Motility Medications)

Prokinetic agents (domperidone, Motilium®; erythromycin; metoclopramide; Maxolon®) can help food move through the gastro-intestinal tract more quickly. They can increase the tone of the lower oesophageal sphincter, increase peristalsis in the oesophagus and hasten stomach-emptying.

- Prokinetics (motility medications) can be affected by some medications. Do not give at the same time as other medications unless specifically advised by your doctor.

## Over-the-Counter Analgesia

With the amount of pain some infants and children have with their reflux, there are times they may need further pain relief. Paracetamol (Panadol® and ibuprofen, Nurofen®) are readily available, but should still be used with caution. It is important to use them as directed, and not for longer than forty-eight hours unless advised by a doctor.

Paracetamol can be used in children from the age of one month, while ibuprofen can be used from the age of three months. Ibuprofen should be used with caution if there is a previous history of gastrointestinal bleeding, ulcers or asthma. Ibuprofen is more likely to upset your child's tummy than paracetamol and should be taken after food. Check with your doctor or pharmacist if you have any concerns.

## Guide to Giving Medication

When medication is prescribed for your child, some things you might like to find out are:

- what the medication is and what it has been prescribed for
- what the dose is
- when and how it should be given
- whether it should be given with food or on an empty stomach (and if with food, whether it matters what food is used)
- how long it can take before you notice any effect/s from the medication
- how it should be stored (e.g. in refrigerator, away from light)
- what the possible side effects are, and what you should do if you notice any
- if there are any special instructions e.g. if it can be crushed, if it has a short use-by date

- what you should do if a dose is missed for any reason (or your child vomits after you give the medication).

*"We were told not to add medicine to a child's formula in case they don't drink it all."*

Talk to your child's doctor or pharmacist about any concerns, and ask for clarification if you are unsure about the dosage, instructions or any details. Ask your pharmacist about any devices that will help you give medication to your child (e.g. Medi-Bottle™).

*"A medication chart can avoid confusion, especially if more than one person is giving medication. Also, it's a good record of when the last dose was given as it's not always easy to remember."*

## Reducing Medicine Costs

Medications, along with doctor's appointments and other treatments, can be expensive. Some of the suggestions listed below may help you reduce your medication costs:

- Pharmaceutical Benefits Scheme (PBS) Safety Net: The PBS provides Australians with affordable access to many prescription medicines. If you or your family reach the PBS Safety Net threshold, you can apply for a PBS safety net card. Your PBS medicine may then be less expensive or free for the rest of the calendar year. Talk to your pharmacist, Medicare Australia, or go to www.pbs.gov.au for further information. For specific information on the PBS call the PBS Information Line 1800 020 613.

*"I use the same pharmacy for our prescription medications, and they let me know when we reach the safety net threshold (because we have a Health Care Card, our medications are then free).*

*It's easier than keeping records or getting printouts from each pharmacy."*

- Health Care Cards (HCC) can reduce the cost of medication under the PBS. You may be entitled to a HCC if, for example, your child requires additional care and attention or you are on a low income. Contact Centrelink for further information.

*"We found out we could get a Health Care Card and we saved heaps of money on our children's medicines and formula . . . Also, I got a printout of all medicines purchased from our pharmacy and I've sent in a claim [to Medicare]."* Tania

- Generic medicines generally cost less than brand-name medications, but have the same active ingredients and are made to the same standards. Ask your doctor or pharmacist if there are suitable, less expensive versions of your child's medicine.
- Some over-the-counter medicines are available on prescription (e.g. Mylanta®, Panamax® tablets/mixture, Movicol®). Buying on prescription may be cheaper because of the PBS (particularly if you have a Health Care Card) and it can help you reach the PBS Safety Net threshold faster.
- Ensure over-the-counter medicines are suitable for your child before buying; talk to your doctor or pharmacist first. These medicines can be expensive, do not count towards the PBS Safety Net limit, and may not benefit your child in any way. Some may interact with your child's prescription medicine or cause side effects, and many liquid medicines contain added colours, flavours and sometimes alcohol.

- If your child is prescribed a non-PBS medicine, some of its cost may be claimable on your private health insurance if you have 'extras' cover.
- It may cost less if you can get medication in a different strength (e.g. if your child takes two ten-milligram medicine and it is available in twenty milligrams, a prescription for the higher strength can mean fewer prescriptions and may be easier to administer). Ask your doctor if this applies in your situation.
- Authority prescriptions: if your child needs more medicine than normal, your doctor may be able to provide an authority prescription under the PBS so you can buy extra medicine for the cost of a standard prescription. This saves money on fewer prescriptions, and fewer doctor/pharmacy visits to get prescriptions.

*"My GP rang Canberra and got a script for us for Alex so we are getting three boxes for the price of one . . . now we have a Health Care Card it is even cheaper." Sharon*

- Do not buy medicine (including prescription medicine) before you need it. It can go out of date quickly, or the doctor may change your child's medicine, which can end up costing you more.
- Home medication reviews can be organised by specially qualified pharmacists. If your child has been taking medication for a while, talk to your doctor or pharmacist about this. It is important for your child's health, but may also save you money.
- Pharmacies vary in prices quite considerably, so shop around for the best price. If considering buying medicine online, beware of the potential hazards and talk to your doctor or pharmacist regarding this.

## Weaning from Medication

Talk to your doctor about how and when your child should be weaned from medication. Just as there are lots of different doses and combinations of medication used to treat reflux in children, there are lots of different ways of taking children off them. Some doctors prefer to stop them suddenly, while others gradually reduce the dose. As with everything else, it can be a matter of trial and error, so be guided by your doctor. Often the best time to try is when your child has been stable for a month or more, and there are no factors likely to cause problems (e.g. teething).

Not all attempts at weaning are successful, but unsuccessful attempts can help confirm you are giving your child medication for good reason. Even if weaning has been successful, your child may occasionally need medication on a temporary basis (e.g. if reflux flares while they are teething or under stress).

*"We tried a lower dose [of medication] at seven months which he seemed to tolerate, so we stopped it, but after ten days . . . he was screaming, not eating or sleeping so we put him back on his medication . . . A few weeks later he was back to being a happy baby!" Mel*

*"Chloe refused her medication just before she turned one. She didn't seem to be in any pain or discomfort and our paediatric gastroenterologist gave her the all-clear." Ula-Jane*

# 10

# Complementary Medicine

> While some natural therapies are covered in this chapter, there are many other therapies that may help with reflux. Please talk to a qualified health practitioner for further information.

There are many different therapies that are considered complementary, natural or 'alternative' in Australia at the moment, such as naturopathy, osteopathy, chiropractics and massage.

Many families use these therapies as a means to help their child with reflux, while other families choose not to. Some may use complementary medicines in conjunction with medication, while others use them instead of. There are many different opinions on this subject, and as with any treatment, what works for one child may not work for another. Some families have amazing success with a particular therapy, while others may not.

Complementary medicines are not for everyone. Do not feel obliged to try a therapy if you feel uncomfortable, no matter how insistent family, friends or acquaintances may be. If you do feel comfortable with the idea of using one or more of these therapies, it is important you do some research and find well-respected, qualified practitioners (ask family or friends as they may know someone they can recommend). Check that therapists are registered with their professional body, and ask about their experience and success rate with infants or children who have reflux. Find out what to expect from the treatments, how many there should be, and what the estimated total cost will be. (Some therapies can be claimed on health insurance, while others cannot, so check with your insurance company before starting.) While offering reassurance that the therapist is well qualified and will offer safe treatment to your child, this does not guarantee the therapy's effectiveness.

It is important to realise that not all natural therapies are necessarily safe. Some can be dangerous if taken or used incorrectly, and some may have side effects. It is advisable to talk to a natural-health practitioner before self-prescribing natural therapies. They can also help you use natural therapies to complement your child's other medications rather than having interactions.

*"Being a natural health practitioner myself I tried many natural therapies to no avail (I'd still use it in other circumstances). I still use natural therapies to manage the side effects we're experiencing with the medication, which is a perfect example of how natural medicine can work hand in hand with orthodox medicine." Kylie Simpson, naturopath*

Some herbal medications can interact with prescription medications, so it is really important to let your doctor know all medications your child takes.

# Biomedical Intervention and Nutrition

Biomedical approaches focus on the fact that health problems are caused by dysfunctions in the body's chemical processes. This approach aims to balance the body's biochemistry so the body can return to a normal level of functioning. Biomedical Intervention focuses on improving gut function, the immune system and liver detoxification processes through dietary intervention, nutritional supplements and avoidance of environmental hazards.

> *"[Our family is doing a] Biomedical Intervention programme . . . we've discovered both girls (and I) are very chemically sensitive . . . Most [foods] still revolve around a small ingredient list, but it's amazing what you can create in the kitchen with such a limited shopping list . . . Lots of changes, all positive, and finally some light at the end of the tunnel." Theresa*

# Bowen Therapy

Bowen Therapy is a non-invasive therapy consisting of small, precise moves that stimulate the connective tissue sheaths to rehydrate and remove toxic cell wastes. It treats the body as a whole and is effective in reducing pain and helping to restore function in a number of conditions. It is based on the recognition that if fascia (connective tissue) is not functioning correctly, it could be the source of many health issues. For more information, go to www.bowen.asn.au.

> *"I took Kiah for Bowen Therapy . . . His reflux has improved heaps; it's just incredible! They use light techniques and Kiah loves it . . ." Lois*

## Chiropractics

Chiropractic treatment aims to heal the whole body. It is based on the belief that disorders of the musculoskeletal system, and particularly the spine, impact on a person's health; and that the body may function better when spinal nerves are less irritated. Childbirth (particularly with instrumental birth) may cause stress to the spine and nervous system, which can interfere with its correct functioning. Some studies suggest that chiropractic adjustments (using gentle, non-invasive techniques) may reduce crying and irritability in some infants.

> *"Clinginess from Jacob has been the misery of my life . . . but since seeing the chiropractor and starting new meds lately he has been a different child and it is amazing."* Bec

## Homeopathy

Homeopathy is based on the idea that 'like cures like', stimulating the body to heal itself. A person's symptoms are treated with substances that will produce the same symptoms in healthy people. These substances are diluted many times over so that the original element cannot be detected.

> *"The homeopath . . . wanted to know how my son behaved when certain things happened and explained there are nine remedies for reflux but you have to match the symptoms with the 'symptoms' of the remedy . . ."* Lois

## Infant Massage

Massage can be relaxing and can help relieve stress. Other benefits include helping with colic, stimulating digestion and improving sleep. Keep strokes long and firm, and focus on the places your child enjoys. While massage for children should always be performed by a parent or close caregiver, you can learn appropriate techniques from a qualified infant-massage instructor. Massage can be a great way of bonding with your child, and can form a positive part of your daily routine.

*"My gorgeous little girl had the most delightful foty-minute baby massage . . . She was the calmest I have ever seen her even whilst awake and she fell asleep with a great big smile before the end. She slept two hours past her next feed." Cate*

## Naturopathy

Naturopathy is a healing system that uses a range of natural treatments such as homeopathy, herbal medicine, nutrition and massage. It supports and stimulates the body's ability to heal itself, and aims to get to the cause of a problem rather than treating symptoms. Where other treatments may focus on controlling symptoms (e.g. vomiting), the naturopath focuses on finding and treating the underlying cause.

A naturopath will take a full medical history as well as diagnostic investigations if necessary, in order to determine the most effective treatment. If using a naturopath, ensure they are a member of an association that recognises their training (e.g. the Australian Traditional Medicine Society).

*"We've been giving Nicky infant acidophilus in every bottle and some homeopathic drops from our naturopath and the last three nights he's finally relaxed enough to sleep almost all night." Lexi*

## Osteopathy

Osteopathy is aimed at restoring the structure and function of the body to a state of balance and health. Cranial osteopathy is a very gentle and safe hands on treatment approach that can help infants and children overcome issues (e.g. unsettledness, feeding and sleeping difficulties, colic, reflux and constipation) that may have developed from the stresses of birth. It may also help children who suffer from ear infections and asthma.

*"[I was told that] birth trauma can have a huge impact . . . apparently it's more common with quick labours or complicated births . . . My osteopath [said] . . . regular manipulation reduces fusion, maintains better health long term and reduces impact stress on other body parts . . . James always comes home more relaxed and sleeps for two hours (that's amazing for him!)." Jessica*

## Other Suggestions

Other therapies may also be used for infants and children with reflux. These may include:

- acupuncture or acupressure
- cranio-sacral therapy.

*"I have a reflux baby, Samuel, who is now nine months old . . . Samuel attended two appointments with a physiotherapist specially trained in [cranio-sacral therapy], and within twenty-four hours I noticed a difference. A week to two weeks after the second treatment he had improved by ninety percent, in my opinion. The physio was quite clear that two treatments were all that was needed and . . . further treatments would not yield further improvement . . . Three weeks [later] I ceased his reflux medication with the blessing of our paediatrician." Samantha*

- kinesiology
- reiki

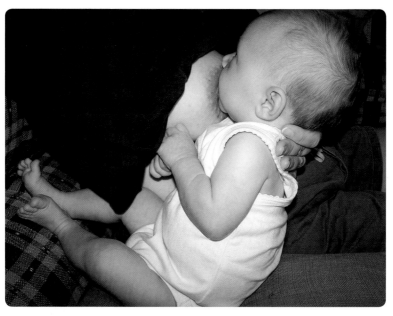

*I often use this position to feed Abbie, with a pillow to give extra support. It keeps her upright and reduces pressure on her tummy.*
**—Bec**

*This position can be soothing for some reflux babies; Abbie really enjoys it.*
**—Bec**

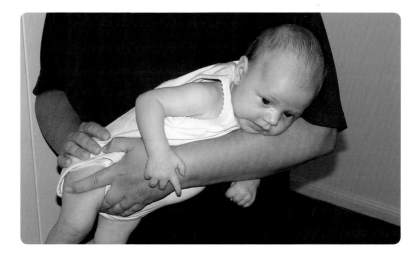

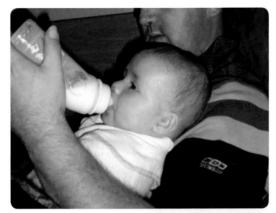

*Daddy Tony found the perfect feeding position for Sumara. It worked really well.*
**–Alana**

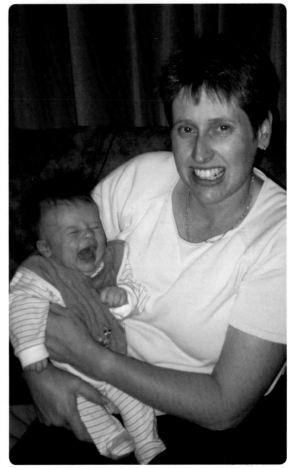

*Before Jorja's food sensitivities were addressed, she was refluxing uncontrollably and I was exhausted.*
**–Trudi**

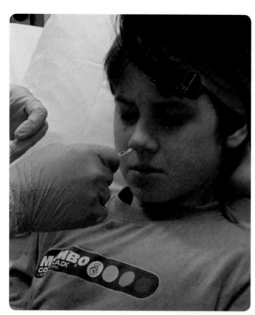

*Anthony (11 years) having the tube inserted for oesophageal manometry.*
*–Glenda*

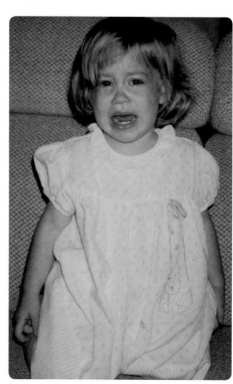

*We didn't know why Natalie was always so miserable, but found out later she had severe reflux.*
*–Glenda*

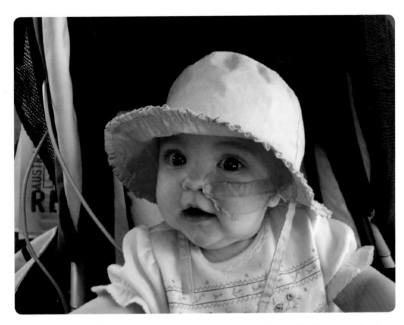

*While I feel really sad about having to give up breastfeeding, we had no other option but to tube feed Emily.*
– **Karen**

*Despite having undiagnosed food and chemical sensitivities, uncontrolled reflux and constipation, Ewan (8½ months) has a ready smile and no weight problems.*
– **Janine**

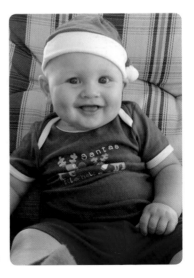

Simple remedies that many families have used include:

- nutritional supplements (e.g. baby teas, chamomile, digestive enzymes, ginger, millet, silica, slippery elm).

*"I'm breastfeeding and started to drink chamomile tea yesterday and can't quite believe the difference. Sacha's vomits are no longer as forceful and she seems more settled." Treacy*

- probiotics (seek medical advice prior to using, particularly in young infants)
- tissue salts for acidity (homeopathic remedies)
- commercial products (e.g. Stomach Calm®, Marina Infant Mixture®).

---

***Important:*** *"If natural or alternative therapies are suggested by other reflux parents, family members or friends, it is very important not to self prescribe or work out dosages, etc. Speak with a therapist experienced in treating reflux infants." Kylie Simpson, naturopath*

---

# 11

# Introduction to Tube Feeding

While feeding issues are common in children with gastro-oesophageal reflux, most are able to be overcome. However, for some infants or children who have reflux, issues such as failure to thrive and feeding difficulties can be so severe or persistent it may make it both helpful and worthwhile to consider tube feeding. This is where a tube is inserted, so that liquid food and sometimes medications can be provided directly into the stomach or intestine.

### If Tube Feeding is Being Considered for Your Child
While tube feeding may benefit your child and your family enormously, the decision to go ahead with it may not be easy. You may be reluctant to accept tube feeding for your child, even if oral feeding is a difficult and upsetting experience. You may have concerns about your child eating normally, or you may feel you have not tried hard enough. You may agree to tube feeding when you feel you have tried all other options, or you may feel relief that your child's feeding issues have been recognised and are being taken seriously. Having information on tube feeding and its benefits and drawbacks can help your family enormously, and can help you make an informed decision.

There are several different types of tubes, and the type chosen for your child will depend on factors such as the reason it is needed, how long it is expected to be used and personal preference. They are named by where they are inserted into the body (e.g. mouth, nose, stomach or intestine), and where the tubing ends (e.g. stomach or intestine). The most common types are nasogastric (NG) and percutaneous endoscopic gastrostomy (PEG) tubes, although tubes can also be positioned to end in the jejunum (the second section of the small intestine) rather than the stomach, if necessary.

An NG tube is inserted into the nose, down the throat and oesophagus and into the stomach, and then taped in place across the cheek area. This option may be used when tube feeding is needed for a short period of time. A PEG tube is inserted through the skin and abdominal wall, directly into the stomach, with its position being determined using an endoscope. The device is then placed in the stomach, with the length of tubing coming out of the body at that site. This type is sometimes referred to as a gastrostomy tube (or G-tube). PEG tubes are sometimes changed to a low-profile device called a 'button' after the site has healed, as this sits very low on the skin. These buttons tend to be hidden from view while your child has a shirt on and are less likely to get pulled on if your child is active. When feeds are given through a button, a tube is attached (so that it is similar to a PEG), and then removed when the feed is completed.

The amount and type of feeds your child has is determined by the doctors and dietitian, according to what best suits your child and family situation, and the position of the tube (whether it goes into their stomach or their intestine). Feeds may be given as a bolus (over a short period of time), continuous (throughout the day at a slow rate, usually through a feeding pump), overnight (often as a way of supplementing feeds), or a combination. The schedule will be adjusted if your child also eats by mouth.

Tube-feeding can offer your child nutritional benefits, with resulting weight gain, growth and development. It can offer validation to your family that there are serious issues resulting from your child's reflux, relief from the pressure of trying to feed your child, and the opportunity to focus on enjoying your child and family. You may find, just as many other families have done, that you would have considered tube feeding earlier had you known how beneficial it would be.

There may also be disadvantages. Emotionally, you may feel like you failed or gave up too quickly, and you may wish you had persevered with oral feeding. Tube feeding itself can be a source of added stress, and there may be issues such as attending to feeds overnight. You may also view tube-feeding as abnormal and this can reinforce feelings of inadequacy, and isolation from other families.

*"Mackenzie had a NG tube from seven weeks, he wasn't putting on weight and was projectile vomiting everything so we didn't have a choice . . . It really did help his reflux, and he was happier with the tube than without . . . The bag with the formula needed to be filled four hourly (he was on twenty-four-hour continuous feeds) so thru the night we would set our alarm so we could fill it up before it ran out . . . This was exhausting, not only waking to the baby but also to the bag! The only advantages were that he really didn't reflux much on the tube when it was continuous feeds and we put all his med[ication]s down it so didn't have the battle. As a result he did settle better and started to develop as the day was not spent screaming in pain for twenty plus hours . . ." Carolyn*

While the major difference with your child is that they are getting some or all of their nutrition through a tube, there are many factors to consider. You need to be taught how to perform tube feeds and care for the tube and insertion site, as well as how to operate the pump if necessary. It is essential that you are taught how to cope with any issues that may arise, and also when to call the doctor or nurse involved in your child's care.

It is also important you are given access to the necessary supplies and ongoing support from speech pathologists, occupational therapists, dietitians, and nurses. Support groups can provide emotional support, and can help put you in touch with other tube feeding families. Centrelink may offer further benefits – you may be eligible for Carer Allowance and other support payments, and their social workers can provide additional assistance.

*"When Emma had her NG tube inserted, we went home with all the necessary equipment and started giving her bolus feeds during the day, and a long overnight feed where the pump automatically pumped in the remainder of her formula . . . We learned tricks along the way to reduce air bubbles in the tubes – making sure to fill the chamber up a bit prior to pumping any milk through the lines before it gets connected, flicking the tube to help all the miniscule bubbles become large enough ones that you can help move out of the tube, etc." Theresa*

# 12

# Introduction to Anti-Reflux Surgery

Most reflux in children is able to be controlled by non-surgical methods (e.g. lifestyle changes, medications, dietary modifications and/or natural therapies), but sometimes these treatments are just not enough. Surgery may be necessary for some children, though it is generally done as a last resort, and like other reflux treatments, is not a cure. It can be an agonising decision for any parent to make, even if it seems to be the only option, and talking to other parents who have been in that position can be extremely helpful.

If your doctor decides that surgery may be an option, your child will be referred to a paediatric surgeon. There may be routine tests that have to be undertaken to not only confirm that reflux is the issue, but to determine whether surgery is an option. Each doctor will have their own protocol, and will also assess each case individually. The paediatric surgeon will review all the information available, discuss all the issues with you and make the decision as to whether surgery is indicated.

Do not be afraid to make an appointment with the surgeon. Making an appointment for a consultation does not automatically mean your child will have the surgery. It can be helpful to get another medical opinion and raise a lot of your concerns early on.

There are general guidelines used to determine suitability for surgery, though they may vary between surgeons, and on a case-by-case basis. Surgery is usually only performed when a child's reflux is severe, or they have persisting complications such as severe oesophagitis, Barrett's oesophagus or strictures; serious respiratory complications; persistent growth issues/failure to thrive; a large hiatus hernia; or chronic pain and poor quality of life.

The type of surgery most commonly performed is a Nissen fundoplication (commonly referred to as a 'fundo'). The surgeon 'wraps' the upper portion of the stomach (called the fundus) around the lower section of the oesophagus in a complete or partial wrap. For each surgery performed, the surgeon aims to make the wrap tight enough to prevent refluxed stomach contents going into the oesophagus, but loose enough to allow food and fluids into the stomach. For this, it is important to find a surgeon who is very experienced as the degree of tightness is an important factor in the success of the surgery.

*"Ella had her fundo at ten months . . . We're very lucky as she had a great recovery and the result was life changing for the whole family." Jo*

The fundoplication is performed under a general anaesthetic, and can be done as an open or laparoscopic procedure. If it is done laparoscopically, the surgeon will use special fibre-optic instruments and monitors to assist. This is occasionally referred to as 'keyhole' surgery, as the surgeon accesses the abdominal area via several small incisions. This can dramatically lessen a child's post-op pain and time spent in hospital compared to when a standard abdominal incision (i.e. open fundoplication) is performed. In addition, scarring is less noticeable. However, an open procedure is sometimes necessary as a result of previous surgery and associated scarring or other complications. There are also occasional times that laparoscopic surgery is converted to an open procedure due to technical difficulties.

---

**Online Research Can Give a False Negative Perspective**
If anti-reflux surgery is suggested or contemplated, many parents research the internet for information. It is important you know that this information does not accurately reflect how successful fundoplications can be, as parents with successful experiences do not need to join support groups or actively participate in chat forums. Consequently, the information you find is often negative and one-sided, which can make the prospect of a fundo even more daunting.

---

Support groups can provide emotional support, and can help put you in touch with families who have faced (or are considering) surgery for their child. They can also provide suggestions that may help in the recovery process.

## Kate

*"It's so difficult to decide about a fundo; it took us ages to agree and then I felt guilty about it. The surgery was far easier than expected, though, and Kate stayed in hospital only one night. She even willingly ate [jelly and fluids], which she'd normally have refused.*

*I was really worried about feeding as it was disastrous the first time, needing speech therapy, etc, and hoped we wouldn't have a repeat of this. Well, it was better, though it was difficult and time consuming at first. After seven weeks, she was eating most of the foods we were, even if a bit slower. She was off all medications by four weeks, and only needed pain relief for a week. She started sleeping through the night by herself, and if she wakes overnight now, she tells us what's wrong (e.g. bad dream) instead of yelling and kicking at us. She also sleeps in one spot, not all over her bed or ending up on the floor because she's so restless.*

*For us it's been the best decision. Life is so much better and I feel that I'm a lot more loving towards Kate now than ever before. Sounds terrible I know. It's also lovely not to hear 'sick in my mouth' a dozen times a day."* Fiona

## Jake

*"Jake (age five years) started grade one this year, just three months post open fundoplication (he has a twelve-centimetre diagonal scar on his tummy) . . . He was very brave during the first few days, and was released from hospital six days later. Our first week at home was a quiet one. Jake's diet was very restricted and he was on what we called 'sloppies' – mashed potato, yoghurt, etc. Just like weaning a baby, we gradually introduced food with more texture. For Jake's sake as well as ours, we made a special 'menu' for him. We thought about all the foods he could eat, then set about finding pictures of them and once the 'menu' was complete, we put it on the fridge. It was good for Jake as he could see what foods he could eat at a glance . . .*

*Jake never complained; he wasn't suffering from any pain and obviously had no reflux. Within two weeks he was his normal self; I actually had to remind him all the time to take it easy*

*as he was just a few weeks out of major surgery. Six weeks post fundo, and Jake was eating all food groups again with ease. You'd never have known he'd had the surgery.*

*Our next hurdle was getting Jake prepared for school, though I think I was more apprehensive than him. He's now been at school for several weeks, and like most children, he's loving it. His fundoplication just three months ago has not held him back in any way. He loves play time, he can run around just like all the other kids, his lunch box is filled with the same foods as all the others, and he's very proud of his scar." Lyndal*

# 13

# Reflux-Related Issues

There are issues that are commonly related to reflux, though the relationship is not always obvious. Some of these issues (e.g. asthma, constipation, ear infections and teething), are discussed in this chapter. Referral to specialists (e.g. respiratory specialist, otolaryngologist ENT specialist) or allied health professionals (e.g. dentist) may sometimes be necessary.

## Asthma

Children with reflux also commonly suffer from asthma, though the connection between the two conditions is not fully understood. In asthma, the small airways in the lungs swell, the muscles contract (or spasm) and the airways can make more mucous, so less air flows through them. This can produce a coarse whistling sound associated with breathing (wheezing), coughing (moist or dry) and shortness of breath. You may also notice other signs such as difficulty feeding (it may be too hard to feed, swallow and breathe), and being less active than usual.

*"Asthma occurs in children after the age of eighteen months when the small airways have enough muscle in them to go into spasm, causing asthma symptoms. Before that age, breathing difficulties in young infants may be due to a virus, infection or*

151

*aspiration (food or stomach contents breathed into the lung air-*
*ways)." Dr Heidi Webster, paediatrician.*

Some children can have silent reflux that presents with asthma, with no obvious signs of reflux (e.g. regurgitation). Their asthma can be difficult to control, especially if reflux is not suspected and treated as a contributing factor. However, it can be complicated, as simply treating reflux does not necessarily improve asthma symptoms, reduce the need for asthma medication or improve lung function, and a referral to a paediatric respiratory specialist may be warranted.

Some researchers believe that reflux may trigger asthma, either directly by refluxing stomach contents into the airways, causing irritation and swelling; or indirectly by stimulating nerve endings, causing muscle spasm. Others believe asthma may also trigger reflux, perhaps by the change in chest pressure from coughing or wheezing. (It is probable that both mechanisms operate in many patients.) Additionally, some asthma medications can relax the oesophagus, potentially triggering reflux.

*"We have found a definite link between asthma and reflux . . .*
*I have also found . . . he didn't need his asthma medications*
*while the reflux was under control." Lyndal*

Reflux and asthma have some similar triggers as well, such as exposure to allergens, viral infections (e.g. common colds, cigarette smoke and exercise), which can complicate matters. Additionally, both asthma and reflux can be associated with throat or chest infections, triggering further reflux and asthma, and it can sometimes be a difficult cycle to break.

As with reflux, there is a variety of ways children with asthma can be treated. Treatments may involve avoiding triggers that bring on asthma symptoms, treating reflux, using asthma medications and controlling allergies. Children with asthma require regular medical reviews.

*If you are ever concerned about your child's breathing, it is important to seek medical advice.*

## Bowel Disturbances

Bowel disturbances, both constipation and diarrhoea, seem to be quite common in children who also have reflux. There can be many reasons for this, such as side effects of their medication, feeding issues (e.g. feeding difficulties/refusal, comfort feeding, overfeeding, excess foremilk), underlying conditions e.g. food sensitivities, inflammatory conditions or motility (movement through the gut) problems, malabsorption of food and infection. Even a lack of fluids due to excessive vomiting and using thickened feeds can contribute to constipation.

Your child may be uncomfortable and suffer from abdominal pain and wind, and their reflux, feeding, sleeping, growth and behaviour can all be affected. How the issue is managed will depend on factors such as the age of your child, the cause of the problem, how long it has been an issue and its severity. It may be a matter of managing the condition or treating the underlying issue.

## Constipation

Constipation is defined as difficulty or delay in passing stool (bowel motions). However, it can be quite difficult to tell if your child is constipated and some normal situations can look like constipation, so talk to your doctor if you have any concerns.

Your child may be constipated if they have difficulty or pain when passing a bowel movement, if they have really hard or pebbly motions, or if they pass less than three bowel motions per week. Constipation may also be a problem if your child appears to suffer from diarrhoea, or alternates between diarrhoea and constipation. This can be due to overflow diarrhoea, which your child cannot control as liquid stool higher up the bowel leaks down around the older, hard stool in the lower bowel. Your child may be so used to being constipated that they are not aware of it, and, like reflux, constipation can sometimes be difficult to diagnose. Some children withhold because they realise it hurts, and may even do a little dance routine or hide somewhere in the house to prevent going. These may all be signs of constipation that need to be treated.

It is important the issue is discussed with your child's doctor to determine the most appropriate course of action. Simple remedies that may benefit your child (depending on their age) include increasing their water intake, using fruit juice or puree, gently massaging their lower abdomen, giving relaxing warm baths, gradually introducing more fibre, and in some instances, removing cow's milk from their diet. Older children may also need to be encouraged to sit on the toilet regularly after meals, with rewards offered as incentives.

*"It is important to treat constipation adequately as it can result in chronic constipation and soiling problems in older children if not addressed." Dr Heidi Webster, paediatrician*

*"Many children do not eat sufficient fibre. It is important that they have a high-fibre cereal once daily and a piece of fruit, and the amount they eat should be sufficient to change their motions to 'sausages'. Some children are resistant to eating fibre and some ingenuity is often needed." Professor Terry Bolin, gastroenterologist*

*"Our child nurse told me to give my daughter a deep, warm bath and let her swim, and leave her nappy off for extra time each day to help things move through the gut." Alana*

In some circumstances your child's doctor may also prescribe medication such as stool softeners (e.g. Coloxyl®) or lubricants. In the last couple of years, laxatives such as Lactulose and Movicol® have become more commonly used in infants and children.

If your child's constipation is severe or difficult to treat, referral to a paediatric gastroenterologist may be necessary. More intensive treatments may be required for the small percentage of children whose constipation remains severe despite persistent treatment.

### Diarrhoea

Diarrhoea is the frequent passage of loose, unformed faeces. Whether it is acute or chronic, extra fluids and rehydrating solutions may be required to prevent or correct dehydration, and you should seek medical advice if you have any concerns. Antibiotics and medications for nausea and/or diarrhoea may be prescribed by your child's doctor and underlying conditions may also need to be managed (e.g. removing cow's milk from your child's diet if they are cow's milk allergic). If the diarrhoea is an ongoing issue, a referral to a paediatric gastroenterologist may be necessary.

## ENT (Ear, Nose and Throat) Conditions

Some children with reflux suffer from a variety of ENT issues such as persistent fluid in the middle ear (glue ear), recurrent ear infections, tonsillitis and croup. Reflux may be a contributing factor, even if there are no obvious signs of reflux. It can be associated with swelling of the adenoids, and can also cause irritation and inflammation to the surrounding tissue. This in turn may cause fluid accumulation and infections. Conversely, ENT conditions and their treatments can trigger reflux so it can be a difficult cycle to break. Additionally, stress on your child can lower their immunity, making infection more likely. The issues can be difficult to control, especially if the link between the conditions is not recognised, and referral to a paediatric otolaryngologist (ENT specialist) may be warranted.

*"[Our paediatric gastroenterologist says] a lot of kids with reflux have enlarged adenoids and tonsils. The enlargement is caused by reflux and it's a vicious cycle then because kids with enlarged tissue reflux more which enlarges the tissue even more!" Nelle*

## Ear Infections

Medical studies have shown that many children with glue ear have pepsin (a digestive enzyme from the stomach) in the middle ear, possibly supporting a role of reflux disease as a cause of ear infections. These in turn can potentially affect a child's hearing, speech and social development.

Ear infections can be treated with antibiotics to improve recovery time and prevent complications. Pain relief is generally provided as well, with oral pain medicines and warm compresses to the ear. Recurrent ear infections may warrant a surgical procedure to drain fluid from the middle ear and insert grommets (tiny hollow tubes) to allow air into the middle ear and prevent fluid building up.

*"At nearly three years, Kate has had many infections, several grommets in both ears, and her adenoids out. A few months ago,*

*she had anti-reflux surgery and grommets and she hasn't had an infection since. Our ENT, paediatric gastroenterologist and surgeon all feel her infections were related to reflux, and I'd have to agree . . ." Fiona*

## Tonsillitis

Tonsillitis occurs when the tonsils (areas of lymphoid tissue located on either side of the back of the throat) become infected. Tonsils can become enlarged as a result of chronic infections. Oral pain medication and encouraging fluids can help your child feel more comfortable, and if the infection is bacterial, antibiotics may be prescribed. There are times that tonsils need to be removed surgically (tonsillectomy) (e.g. enlarged tonsils causing obstructive sleep apnoea or recurrent infections). Obstructive sleep apnoea is the most common indication for surgery in infants and children.

> *"Dolly has enlarged tonsils and adenoids and needs to have them removed . . . the ENT and gastroenterologist told me this more than likely was caused by reflux and that the enlarged tonsils and adenoids can cause them to reflux more . . . The gastroenterologist said once she has them out we should find a big difference in her reflux." Sharon*

## Enlarged Adenoids

Adenoids are areas of lymph tissue in the back of the nose. They can become inflamed as a result of reflux. When they are enlarged, they can cause problems like snoring, mouth-breathing and pauses in sleeping (sleep apnoea). They can contribute to ear infections, obstruct breathing through the nose, and can also become chronically infected on their own.

Enlarged adenoids are sometimes removed surgically, generally at the time of tonsillectomy or the insertion of grommets.

*"Once my son's adenoids were removed, his medication [for reflux] worked too, and we had a happy boy!" Nelle*

## Croup

Croup is an inflammation of the larynx (voice box) and trachea (windpipe), which can cause the upper airway to become swollen and narrow. Your child may find it hard to breathe and may have a barking cough. It is often a mild illness, but it can become serious quickly and it is important to take your child to a doctor for assessment. Most cases of croup are caused by a virus, but croup can also be caused by reflux (known as spasmodic croup).

*"[My son] got a lot of croup when his reflux was uncontrolled." Nelle*

Croup can be treated with steroid medication or adrenaline, which is usually quite effective. In more serious situations, admission to hospital may be necessary.

### Chronic Sinus Disease

Children with chronic sinus disease often suffer from reflux, even if they do not display any obvious signs of reflux. When a child does not respond well to medical treatment of their sinusitis, they may show improvement when they are treated for reflux. Treatment depends on whether sinusitis is acute or chronic. Antibiotics are frequently used, as well as antihistamines and nasal sprays (steroid, decongestant or saline). Surgery may occasionally be required for more severe or persistent cases.

*"Jake has had a lot of sinus infections . . . The ENT said the inside of Jake's nose was damaged . . . consistent with burns from the acid coming up." Lyndal*

## Apnoea

Apnoea is a temporary pause in breathing, and can be classed as central (body fails to take a breath), obstructive (obstruction prevents a breath) or mixed (combination of both). As with other conditions, reflux is known to provoke or worsen central and obstructive sleep apnoea, while both types are known to trigger reflux. Treatment depends on the cause and severity of the apnoea. Tonsils and adenoids are occasionally removed or other procedures or medications may be trialled. Sometimes an apnoea monitor may be used.

## Laryngomalacia

Laryngomalacia, an immature or floppy voice box, is the most common cause of stridor (noisy breathing) in infants. It seems to be linked to reflux in some way. The reflux may cause irritation and swelling of the lining of the voice box, which is a common finding in laryngomalacia. Conversely, reflux may be the result not the cause, because of the increased respiratory effort caused by the laryngomalacia. In the majority of cases, laryngomalacia resolves by itself; however, controlling reflux can sometimes help resolve the 'malacia' more quickly. In some cases, surgery to treat the floppy larynx (voice box) is required.

Tracheomalacia is a floppiness of the walls of the trachea (windpipe) and bronchomalacia is a floppiness of the walls of the bronchi (branches of the windpipe). These conditions can also be related to reflux.

## Eosinophilic Oesophagitis

Eosinophilic gastrointestinal disease (EGID) is a group of disorders in which high numbers of eosinophils are found in the gastrointestinal system. Eosinophils are a type of white blood cell involved in the immune response and are often associated with allergic reactions and food intolerances. EGID is confirmed by finding eosinophils in high numbers in gut biopsies.

*Eosinophilic Oesophagitis (EO)* – high numbers of eosinophils are found in the oesophagus

*Eosinophilic Gastritis (EG)* . . . stomach

*Eosinophilic Gastroenteritis (EGE)* . . . stomach and small intestine

*Eosinophilic Colitis (EC)* . . . large intestine

Eosinophilic oesophagitis often (but not always) occurs in families with food and/or environmental allergies. It can present with symptoms that are very similar to those associated with gastro-oesophageal reflux disease, and some children can suffer from both conditions, which can make diagnosis difficult.

Some of the signs and symptoms typical of eosinophilic oesophagitis are vomiting, regurgitation, heartburn, abdominal pain, choking, refusal to feed, difficulty swallowing and nausea. Children with eosinophilic oesophagitis may fail to thrive and may also have food allergies, eczema or asthma.

*"The paediatric gastroenterologist thinks our son has (eosinophilic oesophagitis). We can't feed him anything but pears and rice at this stage as he's reacted to everything else." Carolyn*

Diagnosis of eosinophilic oesophagitis can be difficult. If a food allergy or intolerance is suspected, a food diary may be used. Note should be taken of reactions associated with particular foods, how the food was prepared, how much was eaten and the amount of time that passed between eating that food and the reaction. Allergy testing may be performed (skin prick testing is most useful).

*"Our allergist says it's clear to him that Jacob has eosinophilic oesophagitis . . . skin pricks and patch testing show he has multiple food intolerances and sensitivities . . . and he has allergic rhinitis (inflamed nasal passages)." Bec*

An endoscopy with multiple biopsies of the oesophagus is the only way to confirm the diagnosis. The oesophagus may look abnormal at endoscopy, and biopsies may show increased numbers of eosinophils. Multiple biopsies are needed because the distribution of eosinophils can be patchy. (In view of this patchy nature, the abnormalities could be potentially missed and if the symptoms persist a second endoscopy may be required.)

Eosinophilic oesophagitis may be treated with medications such as oral steroids (e.g. prednisolone–rarely) or inhaled steroids (e.g. fluticasone–taken using a metered dose inhaler or puffer which is swallowed rather than inhaled). Use of antihistamines and Montelukast (a preventative asthma medication) may help symptoms of allergy and asthma but will not affect the eosinophils.

When food allergies are proven, strict avoidance of the problem food is often the preferred treatment. The child and/or breastfeeding mother may need to follow an elimination diet to identify which foods can be tolerated. An elemental formula may be used in bottle-fed infants. (Dietary manipulation must be done with guidance from a paediatric dietitian or paediatrician.)

Reflux medications are sometimes used if reflux has been proven, because reflux can aggravate oesophagitis. However, symptoms of EO do not usually respond to treatment of reflux with acid-suppressing medication.

EO can cause the oesophagus to narrow in some children. Occasionally, these children may need to have their oesophagus dilated during endoscopy (oesophageal dilatation).

## Teeth Issues

### Erosion and Decay

Australian studies have shown that children who have gastro-oesophageal reflux disease are prone to erosion of tooth enamel and may possibly be more susceptible to tooth decay. Any acid left in a child's mouth after they reflux can dissolve the surface layers of tooth enamel. In some circumstances, dental erosion can be the first sign a child has reflux. Reflux can also cause tooth sensitivity and/or bad breath in some children.

> *"The dentist said that Madi's front teeth were so badly decayed [due to acid] that it was like she had had a bottle of juice in her mouth twenty-four hours a day, which she hadn't!" Karen*

Feeding difficulties common to reflux such as frequent feeding and being very fussy (and perhaps only eating sugary or starchy foods) may also be contributing factors. If your child has an oral aversion or hypersensitivity, brushing their teeth may be difficult, which can also increase the risk of decay. Additionally, some medications can reduce the amount and quality of saliva (causing dryness in the mouth). As saliva helps to neutralise acid and rinse the mouth out, this can contribute to decay as well.

Apart from trying to control the reflux, there may be other practical ways to help reduce the risk of erosion or decay. The following ideas have been listed as a guide:

- Try rinsing your older child's mouth with water before cleaning their teeth, to dilute remaining acid in the mouth. Check with your dentist if there are any rinses, mouthwashes or tooth applications that would be appropriate to harden tooth enamel or help neutralise any acid in your child's mouth. Be aware that young children under approximately six years of age cannot rinse effectively and may swallow any product.

- Try to rinse with water after meals several times a day (if your child is old enough to manage) and also after any reflux episodes, to help neutralise the acid and prevent decay. This lessens the time any acid is in contact with teeth.

- Avoid cleaning your child's teeth straight after a reflux episode as it can brush away the softened surface layer of enamel.

- It may also help to smear a small amount of special remineralising paste (e.g. GC Tooth Mousse™) over your child's teeth following any reflux episodes, and also after brushing in the morning and evening with toothpaste. Talk to your child's dentist for further information.

- Always use fluoridated toothpaste that is appropriate for your child's age, and erosion and decay risk, and remineralising paste obtainable from your dentist. Your dentist should be able to advise you about this.

- A power-operated toothbrush may help, especially if your child dislikes toothbrushes; this can allow for a better clean, without too much effort.

- Talk to your dentist about fluoridating your drinking water if you live in an area where fluoride is not added to the water supply.
- Encourage your child to drink water rather than juice or soft drinks which contain high levels of acids.
- If your child has a drink of juice or soft drink, encourage them to have a glass of water afterwards. This may help to dilute any sugars and acids. It is important to dilute fruit juice or cordial with water as much as possible to decrease erosion; however, this may not reduce decay from these drinks. Soft drinks and sports drinks are best restricted.
- Try to encourage your child to drink using a straw, as this may help lessen the chances of decay, especially if drinking juice, soft drinks or other sugary drinks.
- The use of sugar-free chewing gum (by older children) after meals, and at other times of reflux, is recognised to be effective in reducing erosion as it stimulates the natural neutralising effect of saliva. Chewing gum after meals can also reduce episodes of reflux. Talk to your dentist about chewing gum (available through dentists) that can help harden tooth enamel and reverse the effects of early decay.
- Be aware that medications such as vitamin C tablets and some iron supplements are acidic. These medications may be used in children with reflux, as anaemia and iron deficiency can sometimes be an issue. After administration of products such as these, rinse your child's mouth well, particularly if the medication has been chewed.
- Regular dental checkups are really important from the time that your child's first teeth erupt, as this can help

pick up on early signs of decay, and may even show signs of your child's reflux not being under control. *"All children with reflux should see a paediatric dentist rather than a general dentist." Dr Roger Hall*

## Teething

Teething is one factor that is often reported to flare reflux. For some children with reflux, teeth may cut through without any problem at all, but for others it can be a nightmare. If your child's reflux appears to worsen for no apparent reason, it may be worthwhile checking their mouth to see if they are cutting (or losing) teeth. Surprisingly, it can happen with permanent/adult teeth as well as baby teeth.

Even just understanding what caused the flare-up can be helpful, but you may also need to find ways of relieving your child's discomfort. Tips that may help during teething (depending on your child's age and food sensitivities) are listed below. If offering your infant something to chew or suck on, always provide full adult supervision.

- Offer lots of cuddles and attention to comfort and distract your child.
- Offer ice chips wrapped in a handkerchief to suck or chew on.
- Use teething gels with caution as they contain local anaesthetic. They can also flare reflux, so use sparingly.
- A single dose of a paracetamol analgesic given fifteen to twenty minutes before a feed may help your child to eat (and is more effective than teething gels).
- The peak of pain or discomfort from teething generally occurs one to two weeks before the tooth comes through, although a painkiller (analgesic) should only need to be

used for one or two days. Paracetamol is the only analgesic that should be used for teething, and in the dosage recommended on the packaging. Consult your doctor or dentist if your child is very distressed or you have any questions or concerns.

- Provide teething rusks, rings and toys, or offer vegetables (e.g. carrot, washed and cut into large pieces) for your child to chew on. They may be extra soothing if refrigerated. Always provide full supervision.
- Massage your child's gums lightly using a wet finger.
- Offer your child cold foods or drinks.
- Offer natural teething remedies (in conjunction with medical advice).
- Talk to your doctor about increasing any reflux medications temporarily.

Teething and reflux can also cause your infant to drool much more at this time. To reduce their discomfort and irritability, it may help to keep your infant's chin and chest dry by using bibs, changing any wet clothes quickly and applying a barrier cream to protect their skin.

## ALTE

A very small number of infants with GORD may suffer from an apparent life-threatening event (ALTE), which is very frightening for parents to witness. It may be a result of an infant failing to take a breath, or an obstruction preventing a breath, for longer than twenty seconds. The infant can be seen choking, unable to get a breath, changing colour (going blue or pale) and going either floppy or stiff. If you notice your infant displaying any signs of an ALTE, seek urgent medical care, and if necessary, call an ambulance.

Your infant should be seen by a doctor and will usually be admitted to hospital for observation. Investigations may be performed to find a cause if possible, and determine the risks of your infant stopping breathing again. While an ALTE may never happen again, your infant may be sent home with an apnoea monitor, and you may be taught how to resuscitate your child. If reflux is determined to be the cause, treatment and follow-up will be required.

*"At the end of an unsettled day, Sumara stopped breathing and she became dark blue and very stiff. Thankfully my husband resuscitated her, but she was still very limp when the ambulance officers arrived. After tests were run at the hospital, we were given a portable apnoea monitor to use and we completed a Red Cross course in Infant CPR [Cardio-Pulmonary Resuscitation]. We were also taught [all the SIDS and Kids Safe Sleeping recommendations] to help prevent more episodes." Alana*

# 14

# The Reality and Impact of Reflux

Information in this chapter is provided by parents of children with reflux, based on their own experiences, observations and feelings. While this information can help you feel supported and validated, it may also take you on an emotional journey. You may need to prepare yourself for this, particularly if your experience is still new and your emotions raw.

> *"I really appreciated reading everyone's input [in this chapter]. In fact I had tears in my eyes as I read most of it because it brought everything back for me, but also offered a sense of solidarity and affirmation." Felicity Chapman*

> *"[This chapter] hit so close to the bone I just cried and cried but also felt supported in the fact that it's normal to feel this way considering everything we're going through."*

## The Reality of Reflux

It can be overwhelming when your child suffers from reflux, although many people do not understand this. They may think reflux is normal or even trivial, or may think it is 'just a bit of vomiting' or a 'behavioural issue'. Unfortunately, reflux can range in severity enormously, and families can suffer from extreme stress as a result of having a child with reflux. The lack of understanding of reflux and its associated issues means that many families do not receive the support they need. This can make reflux even more difficult to cope with.

*"At least reflux will eventually become manageable, unlike some sicknesses and disabilities. But for that reason it's often brushed off . . . [With other conditions] there is often support or counselling and a period of grieving but most people don't allow us that . . . It's really only other reflux [parents who] understand what we go through."*

Your experience can be a long way from the joy of parenthood. You may go on a seemingly never-ending emotional rollercoaster ride, and along with the feelings of joy and happiness of having a new baby, you may also have emotions such as confusion, inadequacy, frustration, depression and self-pity. You may believe you lack basic parenting skills, and may lose confidence in yourself. You may grieve for the 'normal' healthy baby you dreamed of, and may question why you are in this situation. You may also have enormous guilt for how you feel, and may act in ways you do not like. As well, sheer exhaustion can magnify all your emotions and make them harder to deal with. Ongoing emotional and physical burdens can also leave you suffering from sleep difficulties, hormonal issues, chronic illness and more.

*"We were just in survival mode. There was no time to bond or play games or even feel any joy at having a baby at all. I felt tremendous guilt and still do."*

*"I was so sleep deprived, frustrated and ANGRY at everyone . . . and mostly my hubby, who cruised off to work every day.*

*Oh, how I wished I could leave the house for eight hours and have a good night's sleep."*

*"Every day can be torture with a sleep-deprived baby and mother; the constant doubts and questioning every little thing to try and solve [the] puzzle . . . one of the worst elements of life with a reflux bub is that it is constant – no breaks, just an endurance test 24/7."*

*"Since the first day . . . I have been scrutinised . . . as to whether I have PND, the ability to parent, just plain neurotic . . . [but] I've never walked so many kilometres with a screaming child, where my arms, brain and heart were numb with pain and grief . . . maybe I just wasn't good enough to cope."*

Relationships can suffer, and partners often find it difficult to understand each other's perspective. Older children may not receive the attention they need, with parents too overwhelmed and exhausted to cope. Social isolation can also be a problem, and an outing with your child can just seem too difficult.

*"[My son's] behaviour [or reflux] is hurting us all. I am finding I have nothing left for my husband or beautiful three year old daughter."*

*"No one really understands what we're going through. I've had so many terrible experiences with her screaming and milk refusal that I'm scared to go out in public with Chloe. The more I attend mums' groups the more isolated/resentful I feel as I look at how happy, calm and cooperative all the other babies are, so I end up feeling worse." Ula*

Despite all this, many people do not accept how serious reflux can be or understand how hard it is for your entire family. Demoralising comments or conflicting advice can add to your confusion and perception of failure. When your family is already in survival mode, the lack of support and comments about what you are doing wrong can be devastating. As a way of coping, you may withdraw from your family and friends at a time you may desperately need all the support, understanding and help you can get.

> *"I've been trying . . . to not talk about it all anymore, as every time I do, I just feel completely dismissed and unheard. I'm spending most of my days trying to analyse my child's symptoms, and the rest of it feeling neurotic and very lacking in confidence as a mother."*

> *"We stopped complaining . . . because we grew tired of hearing 'it's only colic' . . . and being made to feel even more of a failure as a parent . . ." Ula*

You may feel you should be able to cope, simply because everyone expects you to. You may pretend you are coping as a way of dealing with the trauma, and you may be reluctant to let your family and friends help (or even admit you need it). You may start to doubt yourself and play 'mind games', with different scenarios going around in your head. "Maybe it's not as bad as I think!", "Maybe this really is normal and it's just me!", "Maybe I'm doing it all wrong", "Maybe I'm just not meant to be a parent!" are all very common thoughts. It is important you know that even if you are struggling to cope, it does not mean you are failing. Children with reflux can have very high needs, and caring for them can be overwhelming.

> *"It is the most overwhelming experience to go through [with] your child screaming constantly, with no end in sight, and with*

*nothing but confusing and often belittling advice from [people].*
*The constant self-doubt I think was the most crippling and*
*exhausting thing."*

*"Our little boy . . . was/is a nightmare . . . We have been to sev-*
*eral doctors, paediatricians, osteopaths, naturopaths, lactation*
*consultants and have invested in battery-operated swings,*
*pouches . . . prams, sleeping hammocks and who knows what*
*else. Although life is much easier than those nightmarish first*
*few months of almost no sleep and a baby that cried for hours*
*on end, life is still not a bed of roses and there are often days*
*where I still jump in the shower to have a good cry."*

## Carer Stress

It is recognised that carers can be subjected to extreme stress
over long periods of time because of the demands placed on
them; however, it may not be recognised that caring for a child
with reflux can put parents in that position. Even if you desperately seek emotional and/or practical support, you and your
child's suffering may be trivialised because reflux is frequently
thought to be a trivial issue.

*"We took [our baby] in [to hospital] as he spent pretty much all*
*weekend screaming in pain . . . The [doctor said] . . . there is no*
*such thing as reflux and some babies scream 24/7. I just cried*
*. . . Needless to say I'm feeling very tired and stressed and down*
*. . . I've left [my baby] in overnight as . . . my husband and I*
*are at the end of our emotional/mental strings." Lexi*

*"I know the mental cartwheels we do just to exist another day*
*in the middle of reflux hell. It was almost a relief when I realised*
*I couldn't take any more."*

Chances are that you need to be taken seriously, need to be listened to, and need to know you are believed. There is a toll from extreme chronic stress (e.g. health issues, depression, relationship problems), and even the risk of child abuse. These issues need to be recognised, and practical help and emotional support provided. This may help you cope, and it may also reduce the long-term cost to society.

## Living with Reflux: Ethan and Tyler

*From the perspective of Felicity Chapman, social worker, counsellor, reflux parent and founder of Mothers Be Heard (www.mothersbeheard.com)*

> *Reflux is a four-letter word to me. It means torturous sleep deprivation, constant mess, endless washing, numbing exhaustion, and relentless crying – sometimes not just from the baby!*
>
> *While my two wonderful boys are now happy and energetic, with no sign of the havoc reflux caused, I can recall those moments of pure desperation as if it were yesterday. Both vomited in large volumes and 'silently' refluxed (sounded like gulping), were excessively irritable, fed and slept poorly. Bibs were simply mandatory and sleep was a precious commodity.*
>
> *No health professional suggested Ethan's distress might be because of reflux, and Tyler [my second child] was four months old when he was finally diagnosed. It helped that he projectile vomited in front of the doctor! Until then, I hadn't really felt believed by professionals or family and friends. A lot of what happens with reflux happens behind closed doors and in the dead of the night, and that was the most difficult aspect for me.*
>
> *The doctor started Tyler on Losec and gave me a reflux pamphlet [written by the hospital where both boys were delivered]. Losec helped a little, but the questions were obvious: why wasn't*

*I given this information when Ethan was a baby? Why was there no reference to GOR on many parenting sites? Why hadn't any child-health nurse or midwife told me about the possibility of GOR and that there is a gastroenterology nurse at the hospital where they were born?*

## The Impact

*As a social worker, I think of how GOR can impact the individual. It can have an effect on a parent's psychological, behavioural, emotional, physical and social wellbeing. Likewise, I believe that public perception, the quality of professional intervention, and the degree to which parents are supported, can have a huge impact on how they experience GOR.*

*Sleep deprivation, lack of information and practical support, the way people minimised the experience of GOR by suggesting that all babies fuss a bit, the fact that our babies were healthy and didn't seem to get distressed when people visited all contributed to feelings of inadequacy, anxiety, thinking that it must just be me, increased intolerance to stress and social isolation.*

*I don't think I had Post Natal Depression, but I certainly remember feeling exasperated, crying, and having emotional outbursts. I wouldn't be surprised if studies show a strong correlation between PND and parents dealing with reflux. Of course all of this had an impact on my relationship with my husband and children. I'm blessed with a supportive partner and, while the strain showed in our relationship, mostly we knew we were both just plain spent.*

*Unfortunately, both of us looked liked we were coping when we weren't. Perhaps I needed to swallow my pride and look more frayed; perhaps this image adds weight to the saying 'you can't judge a book by its cover'. Everyone, even the baby, can look healthy and normal but GOR can be a private hell because the ferocity of its blow can often be unleashed when no one else is around.*

*Families dealing with reflux need permission to talk about their reality. They need offers of help instead of waiting for them to ask for help. They need help with the washing, looking after the baby so they can get some much needed respite, getting the dishes out the way, and having meals delivered. Most of all, they need to be believed.*

*Reflux might still be a four-letter word to those who endure it, but there are other four-letter words that are much more uplifting. Words like help, care, RISA, and hope can make the journey a lot more bearable.*

Mothers Be Heard has a website and holds workshops aimed at supporting mothers; especially women who have recently become mothers.

## Relationship Difficulties

Relationship difficulties are common amongst reflux families, and although it is a sensitive topic, it is unfortunately another reality of reflux for some families. When you factor in the issues families face, it makes sense there is often conflict within the family unit.

*"An unhappy baby eventually leads to unhappy parents. This was supposed to be the happiest time of our lives . . . but it had truly brought out the worst in both of us." Ula*

Complete exhaustion and sleep deprivation can hinder communication, especially if you feel overwhelmed, unsupported or helpless. Other factors can also contribute, such as

175

if you and/or your partner feel excluded from the relationship or from your child's care, lack support and understanding from family and friends or feel criticised and judged. There may also be difficulties if either partner feels resentful of the time the other spends with the child or if the other can escape from the pressures of home. You (or your partner) may feel tired and irritable, and simple annoyances can turn into catastrophes!

> *"I really think my marriage is on its last legs unless something changes dramatically. My husband's VERY work focused . . . which leaves me doing everything and making every decision . . . I keep telling him he doesn't listen and that I need more input from him, but it does nothing. I'm now on antidepressants and see a psychiatrist . . . I don't know how much more we can 'talk'. I'm ready to pack up and go . . . Who knows what tomorrow will be like but I can't see it being much different."*

## The Impact on Fathers

Mothers are not necessarily the only ones who struggle to cope. Fathers are not immune from needing help, although the 'macho male image' can make it harder for them to seek support. They may struggle to know how to help while trying to be strong for others to lean on, and may need to be persuaded to talk through their emotions or seek support.

> *"I think we sometimes forget our husbands have stressed along with us with the reflux journey, they stress about the baby and they stress about us being stressed and having to deal with it all day and night while they're at work getting a break. They also don't really have the sounding board and support we have . . ."*
> Donna

*"Those years of trial with our (reflux) kids were for me some of the hardest years of my life – no sleep, unrelenting pressure on my nerves, financial pressure, stress on my marriage, lost friends; the list could go on . . ." Wayne*

## Friendships and Reflux

Friendships are often affected because many people do not understand reflux or the impact it can have. While some friendships survive the strain and may become stronger, others unfortunately do not, no matter how good they are/were. Lack of support and thoughtless comments can add to your stress. Until reflux is recognised and taken seriously, and you are believed, this is likely to continue.

*"Our best friends walked away when we needed them most . . . I can't blame them, I would have walked away too if I could have! It still hurts though, even today! If it had been an 'accepted' condition I'm sure it would have been different. What's worse, they judged us, and accused us of not supporting them when we were in crisis and barely surviving. I don't understand how they thought we could do more." Glenda*

*"How helpless you feel. The friends who you thought were friends turn their back. The help you thought you would get is not there. You wonder what you have done wrong . . . They know about your situation, they all talk about you in mums' group, on how much [your son] is screaming and still you get no help! Why?"*

## Child Abuse/Shaken Baby Syndrome

While child abuse is a very sensitive topic, it is a subject that needs to be discussed because the impact of reflux can also encompass abuse. Tragically, being pushed to the edge is a real issue within the reflux community, and it is important to emphasise that anyone can feel this way if pushed too far. While this section may not be easy to read with its open and honest accounts from parents, it does offer suggestions about how to cope if you feel your anger rising or your control slipping.

> *"[My paediatric gastroenterologist] said that most infants that are harmed by their parents are suffering from reflux. If only they had the help they needed!"*

The issue of abuse also covers shaken baby syndrome (SBS), a severe form of child abuse where the infant or child is seriously injured as a result of being shaken violently. Common triggers for SBS are inconsolable crying in an infant or child, along with exhaustion, stress and frustration in ordinary people. Feeding issues are another common trigger. Given that many reflux families experience these issues, it is not hard to see that reflux could push families over the edge.

While it is not easy to admit to getting close to that edge, some families have been open enough to talk about these issues (names have been withheld). Their insight into this problem is quite startling, but even more startling is that families are often expected to cope without extra support, despite having known risk factors for abuse. Some families are told to leave their baby in their cot and walk away until they feel calm, even though this may seem impossible for parents when they know their child is in pain.

> *"[My baby] was very unsettled . . . and there were days where nothing seemed to work. I . . . felt at the point when I was my lowest that if I shook him (which I never did) or gave him a*

*smack (which I also never did) that he may stop crying . . . being home alone, no support and not knowing where to go or who to ask for help, you feel like you have no other option . . . we all know it will NOT make the baby stop crying but at that point you don't think of anything else . . ."*

*"I can totally understand the total frustration and inability to stop a baby from screaming that would lead a person to shake their own child . . . I have had to walk out . . . and leave [my baby] to scream because I could feel myself want to shake her and make her stop – I am so glad I did walk. I can't imagine what would have happened had I not – that few seconds could have changed my life. You are so sleep deprived, that any decision you make . . . in a second – could go either way. I don't think there is anywhere near the support required to cope with a screaming baby 24/7."*

*"Many times I was tempted to shake or throw my child in frustration as I couldn't stand the shrill, high-pitched screaming any more (my husband once measured it at 114 decibels) . . . I don't know how I got through it; it was a living nightmare. I was so alone . . ."*

It is important you are able to recognise when you are not coping, and that you have some strategies that may help. If you feel your stress levels rising, no matter how difficult it is, it may still be best to put your baby down safely (e.g. in their cot), and give yourself some space. Get some fresh air, call a family member or friend, or listen to soothing music; anything to regain control. Though generally it is better to comfort a reflux child quickly, sometimes it is safer to get some time out even if they are in pain. Do not let it escalate beyond that, and SEEK HELP.

Talk to your doctor and/or child-health nurse, and call a helpline or other resource about how you are feeling; it may be the only way you will get the help you need.

> *"It got to the point yesterday that I just left my son in his cot and put my daughter in her room (the safest place for them) then went downstairs and cried my heart out. Once I started, I was unable to stop. I have had to be strong for them for so long I had forgotten I was only human and had needs too."*

> *"I can remember . . . thinking (in the middle of the night feeling sooo exhausted) that I would do anything to get him to go to sleep . . . One night I had visions of holding him by the legs and banging his head against the cot to get him to stop crying. That was my darkest hour and . . . I knew I needed help. I saw the GP the next day and started antidepressants for PND but I think the long-term sleep deprivation from an unsettled reflux baby . . . was the main contributor that led to my depression."*

Another point to consider is that if your child's persistent crying is stressful to you it is likely to be stressful to others as well. If you use a babysitter it is important they understand reflux, what it is and how it affects your child (and especially that your child is not being naughty). It is important they know the dangers of shaking a child, and also how to try to soothe your child if they become distressed (e.g. keeping them upright, using distraction). They also need to know what NOT to try (e.g. laying your child flat after a feed), and that you will respond immediately should they need you. This unfortunately means that any break you get may not be guaranteed. This can make you feel trapped and more stressed, so other avenues may also need to be explored. It is important to ask for help if you feel you are not coping, and to keep asking until you get some! Admitting you need help is a sign of strength, not weakness.

## Postnatal Depression

While studies seem to be limited, research shows that parents of infants with reflux are more likely to become depressed than other parents. In addition to that, sleeping and feeding problems are very common in reflux children of all ages, and both these issues can affect a mother's mental health. Research also suggests it is possible that many mothers diagnosed with postnatal depression are sleep deprived. If you consider the overwhelming stress that many reflux families are under, combined with a lack of recognition by family, friends and society, it is not surprising many reflux parents struggle with postnatal depression, or symptoms that appear similar.

*"I am really feeling down about it all. I don't know whether it is post-natal depression or just depression caused by having such a challenging baby and going through this the first time. I feel like such a failure even though I know I am being too hard on myself."*

*"As far as PND goes, I think that anyone given the same set of circumstances (lack of sleep/support/understanding of reflux), would get depressed . . . I struggle daily with feeling inadequate/hopeless . . . the guilt is overwhelming . . ."*

*"Two weeks after starting my antidepressants I [noticed it was] the first day I [hadn't] cried or wanted to cry since my son was born. He was five months old. No one really saw my PND as he was so difficult that everyone just thought I was emotional because of that."*

## Financial Impact

In addition to the physical and emotional impact of reflux, the unexpected financial impact can add significantly to your stress. This is not only about doctor's bills or medications; there can be cleaning bills, extra electricity and water bills from all the washing, trialling different therapies, buying books or endless products and services in the bid to find something that helps.

> *"Financially [reflux] can be a burden as we spend a fortune at the pharmacy and are constantly seeing doctors and specialists, then trying naturopaths, osteopaths, homeopaths, etc, as we search for some small miracle to help our baby. Then we have the outlay for the various pouches, most comfortable pram, battery-operated swings, toys and accessories that may give us just ten minutes to throw on a load of washing."* Jules

Some ideas that may help reduce the financial impact of reflux are listed here, with further suggestions listed under the article on resources.

> *"Keep receipts for all your out-of-pocket medical expenses so you can claim them on your tax return if necessary."*

> *"If you live out of town, check if you can claim for travel to specialists. Some health-insurance coverage includes an annual amount for travel." (You may also be entitled to travel and accommodation subsidies arranged through your local hospital.)*

> *"Some doctors will reduce their fees if you explain medical bills are mounting. I once had a doctor take $100 off the bill when I explained our financial situation."* Glenda

*"We used a toy library to provide our daughter with a range of stimulating toys. We found out what interested and distracted her without the expense of buying them all."*

*"Even if family don't understand reflux or what you're going through, they may be more sympathetic to financial strain, so gifts of money at birthday or Christmas to help pay for treatments helps. James' grandmother booked and paid for a month of acupuncture for him . . . I thought it was a great present!"*
*Jessica*

*"Accessing parenting magazines and books at the library can help keep costs down."*

# 15

# Coping with Reflux

## Tips for Coping with Reflux

Caring for children with reflux can be overwhelming. These following tips from parents may help:

- Do not expect to have all the answers from the beginning – it is a steep learning curve, and chances are you did not know much about reflux before you had your child.

- Children with reflux are not born with a manual, and there is generally no right or wrong way to handle a situation. What works for one may not work for another, so it is often a matter of trial and error until you find something that works.

- Accept that you are doing your best, and try not to be too hard on yourself (be realistic with your expectations and limitations). Trying to 'keep up with others' when your child has reflux can add extra stress without benefiting you or your family. Do not feel as though you have to do it all yourself!

*"I put a lot of pressure on myself to be the perfect parent, despite all the issues we faced from reflux. Once I accepted I was doing my best I found I coped much better." Glenda*

- Try to focus on what you feel is going right, not what is going wrong. You are not doing anything wrong; you just may not have worked out the best answers yet.

- Realise your situation is tough; children with reflux can have very high needs, and most people do not understand what you are going through or how to help – this may come out in unhelpful things they say, or by not offering support and help.

- Listen to everyone's advice; however, do what feels right and ensure the choices you make are safe for your child. Discuss any issues or concerns with your doctor.

- Believe in yourself and trust your instincts; reflux is a medical condition and not in your head.

*"Please, don't ever ignore your instincts . . . If I hadn't listened to [mine] . . . [my son] would still be in much pain and I'm sure I'd be in hospital myself by now, after a breakdown. So don't ever feel you're exaggerating or being too precious. No one else is going through what your family is and no one else knows your baby as well as you."*

- Look after yourself – not only are you as important as your child, think about who will be there to look after them if you fall apart!

*"For the really bad days, when I had no energy (or had had no sleep), I had activities (e.g. DVDs, games) hidden away as a treat for my older kids. They were occupied and I got the break I desperately needed."*

- Live in the present. Try not to dwell on the past or waste time worrying about what might happen in the future.
- Try not to be a perfectionist or expect too much from yourself or family members (they may be as stressed and upset as you but may show it differently).
- Remind yourself that this is NOT your fault.
- There are many factors that are reported to flare a child's reflux e.g. teething, illness. Sometimes it can help to know that, so any changes in your child make more sense.
- You can drive yourself crazy trying to figure out why today was better or worse than yesterday ("What did I do?" "What did I eat?" "Maybe if I tried . . .?"). The simple fact is, reflux can be cyclical and some days may be worse than others for reasons you may never know.
- Talk it over. Try not to bottle it up; ring a friend or a support group. It can help to relieve the strain and often helps you to see what you can do about the issue.

*"Groups like MyTime and Good Beginnings provide support to young children and their families."*

- Think about how you might change a stressful situation (e.g. take your child back to the doctor or get help in the home). Accept offers of help if they do actually help you.

*"When you say reflux, people always say 'Oh, is that all?' So now we say OTR (oesophageal tracheal reflux) and they at least try and act supportive."* Alana

- Take one thing at a time. Focus on caring for your child with reflux, your family, and yourself (not necessarily in that order). Take care of the urgent tasks and leave the rest to be done when you have time, or to be done by others (e.g. cleaner, friend).

- Try to ignore comments about how lucky you are that your child's condition is not worse. You know that, but it does not help you cope with the screaming and other issues now!
- Encourage and allow your partner to participate in your child's care.
- Avoid blaming each other for the suffering you are going through. Everything always seems much worse when a child is screaming.
- It may help to accept life as it is so there is some degree of peace of mind, rather than fighting against it and expecting a cure in those children whose reflux continues to be an issue. It may not be fair, but that is the reality.

*"The best advice I was ever given was don't fight it. Once you accept that you can't change it, things will become a whole lot easier." Lyndal*

- Remember that your child with reflux is not being naughty or intentionally difficult; they have a chronic condition and it is not their fault. The same may apply to other children in the family as they may be affected as well.
- Recognise that there will be times you feel more able to cope, and more positive, while other times you may feel quite low and overwhelmed. This is normal.
- Take each day as it comes. Life really can get better, no matter how hard it is right now. Remember, though, that if you are not coping ask for help or seek medical guidance.

*"The doctors said my son would improve when he could sit or was on solids, but he didn't. My dashed hopes made coping even more difficult. It helped when I started focusing on each day as it came rather than looking too far ahead." Glenda*

## Looking After Yourself

You may feel you should totally focus on your child, and may even feel selfish if you take time out to look after yourself. Apart from realising you are important; you need to ponder what would happen if you fell apart, or who would look after your child if that happened. Remember, you are the most important person to your child, and you need to stay healthy for them.

Value yourself and the role you play, and do not feel guilty about any strategies that help you look after yourself. The following suggestions may give you some ideas on achieving this:

- Give yourself rewards and take pride in even the smallest achievement.
- Take some deep breaths of fresh air; go for a walk around the block (while someone minds your child). Calm yourself down and then go back and deal with the situation.

*"Go for a walk if baby won't stop crying; it doesn't seem so loud when you're out." Sharon*

- Try to eat regular, healthy meals.

*"Have lots of healthy snacks ready, as you need to look after yourself too." Sharon*

- Consider using a sling – it may help you get things done while keeping your child upright.

*"Buy a sling that keeps your child upright whilst you do something two-handed." Trudi*

- Roster sleeps (e.g. one copes with your child until a specific time and the other handles the issues for the second shift).
- Try to organise it so you can sleep when/if your child sleeps; switch off your phone and encourage friends to call you before visiting. Do not be afraid to put a note on the front door saying something like "We are sleeping – please do not knock!"
- Try to continue doing activities you enjoy, even if it is difficult.
- Set aside some time each week for relaxation or a simple outing (e.g. shopping or coffee). Plan outings for yourself and your partner (e.g. take a walk, go to a movie) and make yourself go. It may be difficult to make the effort, but can help you feel better.
- Try doing something that can lift your mood; listen to music, get out an old photo album, phone a friend, have a massage or do something silly like blowing bubbles. Sometimes being able to laugh can help relieve the stress.
- Get some regular exercise, if possible.
- Plan an outing with your child (e.g. a walking parents' group or playgroup). This can help you get out of the house, interact with others, and give you a chance to make new friends.
- Accept that your child's behaviour is not the usual behaviour of a child. Knowing this may help you cope when friends tell you about their perfect child. Realise it is

harder for you, and you may not be able to achieve everything they do.

- Get help around the house, or tend to only essential household chores. Only fold nappies when needed or use disposable or fitted nappies. Use a cleaning person or nappy service if possible. Investigate pre-packaged meals or meal delivery.
- Use an online shopping service with home delivery, if one is available.
- Plan and prepare meals on the weekend if you have an opportunity. Knowing what to cook can make a difference. Stock up the freezer with frozen meals, if possible.
- Prepare the evening meal early in the morning so when the afternoon comes around, you are not too tired, stressed or busy to deal with it. Use a slow cooker, if it suits.
- Ask family or friends to supply a home-cooked meal that can be eaten that day, or frozen for later, when they next visit.
- Organise family or friends to babysit for a couple of hours while you go out and have a break. Maybe they would take your other children to the park for a couple of hours so your children can have a break too. If you can, take advantage of your break and look after yourself: have a nap, or take a long, relaxing bath.
- Let your family and friends know how you are feeling, and ask for help. This may be hard to do, but sometimes friends/family will be happy to help if you ask them.

*"Accept ALL offers of help. And (this is the hard one) ask for help. Something I found really difficult, and wish I had done it.*

*My friends tell me now, when I have told them how awful it was, that they never realised, and I should have asked them to help." Jody*

- Accept those offers of help that you feel will be helpful for you and your family.
- Be aware that despite what you might say, some friends and family might not want, or be able, to help. Although this is hard, you cannot change everyone! Focus on you and your family and maintain contact with those family or friends who are supportive and non-judgemental.
- Consider returning to work if you need time out, and to restore your flagging morale.
- Pay someone to babysit or consider putting your children into childcare to give yourself a break. Information about childcare services and government assistance is available from the Child Care Access Hotline. Some families may be eligible for In Home Care.

*"An option for a break and support is In Home Care . . . We have just started to use this service and had our first visit from our carer yesterday. You can use your childcare benefit to help subsidise this, but you can also apply for funding . . ." Karen*

- Talk over your concerns with another reflux parent who understands how you feel. Contact a support group or, if you have internet access, go online as there are a lot of chat groups that may suit.
- Have contact details of support services handy in case you need them; including twenty-four-hour parenting help lines (e.g. *healthdirect Australia*, Lifeline, ParentLine, ParentLink).

- Contact your local doctor, hospital or child-health nurse about accessing support services (e.g. a social worker, psychologist or parental help). If your child has complex care needs, in-home support may be available.

*"During one of my daughter's hospital stays, I was in the depths of despair: I asked to speak with [a social worker]. After some long chats and bucket loads of tears they were able to get some physical help at home for me [with a parent aide]. Only two hours one day a week, but boy did I look forward to that day. It REALLY is worth a try." Jo*

- Find a local doctor you feel comfortable and confident with, and who you can talk to, so that you can talk about all the demands on you.

## To Family and Friends

Just like many parents caring for a child with reflux, you may find it difficult to ask for help, or accept it even if it is offered. You may feel bad you cannot return the help, you may not want others to know you need it, or you may feel you should be able to cope without any help.

Additionally, some well-meaning family/friends have the knack of saying the wrong thing and making it worse! They may think they are helping if they pretend everything is okay; however, this can discourage you from opening up or accepting help.

*"I got told that Jacob was allergic to me when his reflux was so severe as a baby. "Thank you for that" . . . like I don't feel bad enough already." Bec*

*"Going to the new mums' group was unbearable. Chloe was the only baby who'd scream the whole time and refuse feeds and*

*what were supposed to be 'support groups' made me feel a hundred times worse. Our family and friends mainly saw Chloe for short periods; they didn't see her meltdowns and thought we were over-reacting. We felt unsupported and our marriage suffered greatly." Ula-Jane*

Family and/or friends can do a lot to help, and these ideas have been listed as a guide. Show it to family and friends if you wish and talk to them about it. Add suggestions if appropriate, and encourage your family and friends to do the same.

- Be available, and encourage both parents to talk about their day as well as their reality (including feelings, issues and experiences). Avoid presuming you know what their role entails, and try not to pass judgement. Listen to them and believe them.

- Acknowledge their difficult role and provide encouragement and validation to both parents. They may need confirmation they are doing a great job.

- Be aware that lots of people offer advice, much of which is conflicting. Even though the advice may be well meant, it is often confusing, and can make parents feel inadequate. It may be better to offer practical help and/or emotional support.

- Encourage both parents to look after themselves.

- Reassure both parents that asking for or accepting help is a sign of strength, not weakness, and that they should not feel guilty for needing help.

- Many parents grieve for the easier-to-care-for child they did not have, or the experience of parenthood they may be missing out on. Allow them that, if necessary. Also, please do not suggest that they should be grateful for the life of their child and that it could be worse!

- Allow the parents to take breaks from their caring role, either informally or regularly.
- Offer to help the family, rather than waiting for them to ask for help.
- Provide meals the family can either eat now or freeze for later use.
- Prepare healthy snacks for the family.
- Help with any housework (e.g. washing, ironing, cleaning the bathroom). Some parents feel more in control if the house is clean and tidy.
- Encourage the parents to focus on managing on a daily basis, rather than searching for that elusive cure, or focusing on when the reflux will be gone. Try to refrain from telling them their child will outgrow their reflux any day now.
- Isolation is often a big problem, so try to provide companionship. Accompany the family on outings and offer your support; many reflux families find it too difficult to go out.
- Offer to drive them to medical appointments. Some parents can be so exhausted they will cancel a much-needed appointment rather than drive there.
- Offer to attend medical appointments with them.
- Help the family maintain their routine if possible.
- Spend time with older children as they may feel neglected.
- Make a list of things that others could do to help; the parents may not have thought of ways that others can help.
- Do some grocery shopping for them, or check to see if they can get groceries home delivered. Ask them to pre-

pare a list so you can get their groceries when you do your own shopping, or get the essentials you know they will need.

- Find out if their local pharmacy home delivers.
- Organise other services as appropriate, such as a nappy delivery service.
- Try to make helpful comments that show you understand, or would like to. Try not to make comments that help you feel better, as this can undermine any attempts you make to help. While there can be any number of things people say, statements such as "I think you may be overreacting", "I can't see anything wrong with baby", and "You should (or shouldn't) be doing...." are generally not helpful.

*"Mothers' groups [can make you] feel isolated because nobody really understands what you've been through. Or worse, feel judged because everyone tells you that you're doing something wrong which is why your baby is waking/crying/not eating, etc."*
*Jules*

## Benefits of Support Groups

Support groups can provide enormous benefits. The understanding and support they can provide, along with management suggestions, may help you cope. Talking to other parents of children with reflux can make all the difference.

*"Many times I have posted [to the reflux group] because I had just had enough and needed to vent . . . Not only do we . . . deal with the reflux itself, but our isolation from 'normal' people who just don't get it . . . financial stress from the extra pressure of medical costs . . . fragile marriages, guilt . . . resentment, anger,*

*frustration and on it goes . . . [The group] saved me from a life I don't even want to think about. A kind word, lots of under-standing . . . all just as valuable as the practical knowledge."* Jody

*"[When I joined a support group] I was so relieved to see there were so many experiences that were similar to ours, and . . . I think it helped me to realise that it wasn't just me, or something that I was doing! I learnt so much when I first joined . . . and feel it gave me the strength and knowledge to keep fighting for my children. I also was able to see how serious reflux could be and also what effects not treating it could have."* Karen

## Positive Consequences of Severe Reflux

Even though it may not seem possible, parents often report pos-itive consequences of reflux, such as learning to be more compassionate and less judgemental, recognising strength and resilience they did not know they had, learning not to take any-thing (or anyone) for granted, and finding new friendships. Parents often find they learn to look for the positive in every sit-uation, and that reflux teaches them that it is possible to grow and thrive through adversity. They may also report benefits for their children.

*"There are still many days I doubt myself as a person and mother. What gets me through is knowing I've become a better person from having a reflux child. It would have been so easy for me if I had a quiet baby to ignore, and get on with my busy life fulfilling my dreams . . . What my reflux babies have taught me and are still teaching me is that I must stop and enjoy the moment . . ."* Caterina

*"The reflux journey brings out qualities in us that we need even if we didn't know they were there. When I'm having bad days with the kids, I try to remind myself that some amazing benefits have come of it."* Theresa

*"The 'coming' of the second child was an anxious time [after having a child with reflux] but we were pleasantly surprised and relieved he did not present with reflux but mild food intolerances which were easier to cope with. Hence, the decision for the third was easy . . . our third son is a feeding and sleeping contented bundle of joy (yes, that urban legend, textbook child does exist). All good things come in threes . . . and although the third child is the easiest, it was the first who taught us the most and made us stronger."* Tennille

## Resources

There are many resources available, but you may be too overwhelmed with the stresses of reflux to find them. Your doctor or child-health nurse may be able to guide you or refer you to appropriate services, and your local hospital, or state or territory's health department may be able to provide further assistance.

You may also find services in parenting books, telephone directories and on the internet. Some government websites that may help are www.australia.gov.au (provides links to Australian Government Departments and Agencies), www.community. gov.au (provides access to online services and information) and www.mychild.gov.au.

Keep in mind that services and details can change over time. Contact the relevant service providers for up-to-date information regarding the assistance you may be entitled to.

*"Hospital social workers . . . are great and can usually provide some support as well as putting you in touch with other counselling and support services. Your GP should also be able to organise some counselling for you . . . [We now have] a community nurse who comes to visit . . ." Karen*

*"I talked to a social worker from Centrelink. She provided support and gave me information on community services and Centrelink payments we were eligible for."*

*"Many reflux families are eligible for Carer Allowance (it isn't income tested). Not only does it help a great deal with ongoing medical costs, it provided the validation I needed that my child had very high needs!"*

*"If you aren't eligible for Carer Allowance, you may still qualify for a Health Care Card. This makes prescriptions and prescription formulas much cheaper." Janine*

*"We registered all of our family members for the Medicare Safety Net. Now we've reached the threshold, our Medicare rebate is higher and our doctor visits cost less."*

*"I'm bordering on PND . . . [my GP] suggested a mental health assessment to get a Medicare-rebated psychologist . . . it makes the help more accessible and affordable."*

Reflux Infants Support Association (RISA) Inc
www.reflux.org.au

# 16

# Personal Stories

The following stories have been provided by families whose lives have been affected by reflux. Even though your journey is likely to be different, you may identify with some of the experiences and emotions they have shared. You may also like to consider writing your story at some stage, as doing this can be comforting and may even be therapeutic.

## Celina

*Celina cried from the time she was born and I was exhausted, even in hospital. She soon started vomiting; I was in tears all the time and had no idea what I was doing wrong. I 'jokingly' told everyone I'd throw her out the window if it wasn't for the security screens – but deep down it was how I felt at times.*

*The GP shattered my morale by telling me I was underfeeding her. Fortunately, my child-health nurse knew there was something wrong, and sent me to the hospital. The doctors there diagnosed Celina with reflux. Antacids and thickeners didn't help, and nor did Zantac®, and she was eventually admitted to hospital for observation (she'd take the breast, but then scream and refuse for hours).*

*The paediatrician said to give her formula as she'd lost*

*weight, but I was determined to keep breastfeeding. Unfortunately, she'd cry as soon as I undid my shirt. I was again demoralised, feeling rejected by my own daughter – I couldn't do 'the most natural thing in the world'. I found out later that feeding issues and breast refusal were common with reflux; my baby associated the breast with pain. Thickened formula helped but only for three days. She started crying at night with a different pain so we changed formulas many times trying to find one that helped (not knowing how many we'd try or how much money we'd waste before realising nothing does).*

*Through all this my husband started a new job, and was away most of the time. I felt like I was going to break. I was alone in a new town [we'd moved when Celina was six weeks old] and had no one to help. Some days I didn't shower and only ate one meal.*

*The child-health nurse referred us to an early-parenting centre. We spent a week there getting her to sleep in her cot (which she now does). Their paediatrician changed her medicine to Nexium, and suggested Neocate (an elemental formula). It took longer than I expected to see a difference with the medicine but it did help. The Neocate made no difference, so we ended up back on a HA formula. She still doesn't sleep for long but can be settled without a bottle or crying – I think my love of her dummy is causing some of those issues.*

***Update:*** *Celina is now eleven months old. She's still medicated, despite trying to wean her recently – but she no longer screams at every meal. She also still vomits, though not like she used to. She sleeps well at night, and when I finally got the courage to see if she'd sleep without the dummy was amazed that she did. She also transitioned to solids well, although certain foods do trigger vomiting.*

*I know the road is long, but I'm living proof that things do get better and being a mum is so rewarding now.*
  *Deborah*

# Daniel

*Within a week of being born, Daniel became what everyone described as colicky, windy and "just a difficult baby". By six weeks he became more unsettled, crying for six to eight hours every day before falling asleep exhausted at five pm, sleeping til ten pm when it would start all over again. He never slept longer than twenty minutes in the day and would wake screaming. I told myself everything would settle down when he was a little older, as it did with his sister . . .*

*The screaming continued but he was feeding well and gaining weight (even though he was born at 97th percentile and had dropped to 50th) so health nurses and doctors told me he was perfectly healthy and instead directed everything at me. I heard it all. My milk letdown was too fast. He was gulping air. I needed to let him cry. Was I burping him effectively? Was I feeding him too often? I twisted myself inside out trying to do every little thing "right" but everything just got worse. I stopped going out, I hated getting together with other mothers. I felt that everything was too hard and fell into depression. I look back now and don't know how I never hurt him because believe me; I thought about it a lot. If only I had RISA then!*

*The screaming continued until at four months he began to totally refuse breastfeeds. Finally, one day I was crying and my two year old was crying while I was trying to feed him. It was about as bad as I think it can get as far as not coping. I rang the health line (for the fiftieth time) and told them I was ready to* snap. *The nurse on the phone told me to get out of the house and away from the screaming and I informed her that I was standing in our backyard. That phone call finally got the ball rolling.*

*Daniel was diagnosed with silent reflux and was put on [medication] which worked well for a week. His medication was changed . . . and he improved dramatically within forty-eight hours. His sleeping improved – he slept during the day and only woke twice at night but he was still a fussy feeder and would usually become very irritable every afternoon. At six months he was weaned from the breast because I had had enough. Things just got worse around five to six months and the screaming started again.*

*This time I was confident enough to tell the ugly truth about what was happening because I KNEW it was not about me and I knew my baby better than anyone. A paed[iatric] gastro[enterologist] suggested we put Dan on Neocate and cut out all dairy foods and booked him in for an endoscopy. After forty-eight hours with his new diet Dan was a completely different baby and no longer required an endoscopy (will keep it in the back of my mind however) . . .*

*Daniel is now ten months old and I still cry, but it is mostly with joy. He is still medicated . . . and off dairy and we just take it one day at a time. Right now our family is in what I call recovery mode and a bad day can still knock the stuffing out of us, but what gives me the greatest pleasure is seeing my gorgeous boy laughing and giggling with his sister and dad . . .*

## Jacob

*"I've written Jacob's story without emotion, for fear of breaking into tears if I tell of the emotional heartbreak we went through day after day, week after week." Bec*

*Jacob cried all the time, fed frequently day and night, and vomited from the beginning. By six weeks, he screamed uncontrollably, never slept and often had small brown spots in his vomit; he soon started vomiting obvious blood and mucous. A paediatrician diagnosed reflux and prescribed Zantac. By ten weeks he was on Zantac and needed antacids before every breastfeed. He still screamed uncontrollably, but the paediatrician said he'd get better. By six months he'd stopped growing properly.*

*At nine months, we moved interstate. He started vomiting large amounts of blood, was thin and gaunt, and started gagging when he was breastfeeding and having solids. He had ulcers on his tongue and a paediatrician started him on Losec. The dose was increased steadily, but at twelve months he only weighed eight kilos.*

*A barium swallow at sixteen months was normal, so we continued with the same medications, going through bottles of Gaviscon a week. At twenty-one months, weighing only nine kilos, Jacob had a pH probe, with his sleep and colic monitored. He refluxed continuously, within normal limits (but took medication the entire time). He woke every half hour overnight and I breastfed him ten to twelve times a day. I changed paediatricians again, still searching for someone who could help. His Losec was increased and he started motility medication; two weeks later he stopped vomiting.*

*A chiropractor at twenty-two months helped with sleep issues and life appeared to be normal for a while. He grew rapidly now he'd stopped vomiting, and at two years Jacob weighed ten kilos. The change in him was amazing, although he still had eczema.*

*We moved again when Jacob was two and a half years old, and our new paediatric gastroenterologist performed an endoscopy. It confirmed moderate/severe reflux and his Losec was increased again. He was once again vomiting through the night. An allergist performed skin pricks and patch-testing which showed Jacob had multiple food intolerances and sensitivities. With help we modified Jacob's diet so he's no longer violent, aggressive or screaming all day and his eczema has disappeared.*

*At four and a half years Jacob is thriving, happy and outgoing and his specialists are happy with his progress. He's now on the 90th percentile for weight and height.*

***Update:*** *At six years Jacob takes Nexium, multiple medications for asthma and allergies, and we've learnt he's anaphylactic to eggs and grass. He also relies on Neocate for most of his nourishment. Whilst he continues to struggle with reflux, food intolerances, and eating/sleeping issues, he enjoys swimming, nippers, Little Athletics and cricket. For the first two and a half years, breastfeeding was my one nice connection with him; the only happy time we had. We have a much closer bond now; he cuddles and kisses, and is an outgoing, stubborn little man. He has a bright future ahead of him and I'm sure he'll achieve whatever he desires.*

*Bec*

## Liam

*Liam was a water baby and I had no pain relief for his birth, but he had great difficulty attaching to the breast and constantly vomited. The nurses said it was normal. I had issues with that; I knew something wasn't right. His cry sounded like a pain cry, and we battled with every feed.*

*They thought I might have postnatal depression – if I didn't, I definitely experienced symptoms when my concerns weren't being heard. I was so relieved when I got a different opinion and Liam was diagnosed with reflux.*

*I was against giving my child medication at six weeks; it was definitely not in my plan, but also knew it was best for Liam. He was more settled and slept and fed better, which allowed me to get some rest and feel human again. Unfortunately, it didn't last. We'd have good periods; then periods where he wouldn't feed or sleep well. At the time I had no idea this was normal for reflux babies.*

*I persisted with breastfeeding for ten weeks until it was so stressful I couldn't do it anymore (it's definitely a two-way process and needs to work for both of you). He started on an elemental formula (EleCare) and the difference in his feeding was amazing. He regurgitated less, slept better and screamed far less at feeds. We confirmed his cow's milk sensitivity and it felt like we had a new baby. I could handle an off day here and there, and felt better within myself. Going back to work three days a week helped too.*

*We slowly introduced dairy at about ten months on our specialist's advice – we trialled this very slowly over a four-week period with success. We didn't notice any signs of cramping or mucous in his faeces so that was good. We then trialled wheat and soy products, one by one, using the same process, and by the time Liam was thirteen months old he could tolerate them in his diet in moderation.*

*It makes me upset and angry that reflux is so under-diagnosed, and parents (in particular first-time mums) are told that things are normal when they themselves sense they're not. I've learnt it's important to trust my judgement and be persistent until I'm happy with what I hear.*

*To anyone reading this, if you have children with reflux, hang in there – things do get better. If you're friends or family, be a support and talk to them as it can be a very long, isolating experience. I know the rollercoaster ride may not truly be over but we can certainly deal with the challenges much better now we're sleeping better and have a better understanding of GORD. I used to be a person who'd rarely ask for help; but I needed to learn. Don't be shy or too brave and ask for help when you need it. It makes all the difference.*

*Belinda*

## Noah

*Noah is four and a half months old and everyone comments on how placid and happy he is. I guess I wanted to start at the good part as there is light at the end of the tunnel.*

*Being the naturopath I am, I made every effort to conceive a healthy baby. I was able to go home four hours after his birth and he slept through his first night, but by the third night, I could no longer feed comfortably, and was advised to return to the hospital. This is where the many opinions became apparent. "Express." "Try and feed." "Burp him." "Don't burp." The lactation consultant helped correct our latching, and I went home. Nights were hourly feeds, and Noah was very unsettled. We went on a rollercoaster of some good feeds then a bad one and I was at the end of my tether.*

*The GP told me it was colic (she'd had a colicky baby and if there was a cure she'd be a millionaire). Things deteriorated and I tried natural medicines, Infacol, Brauer, gripe water. The mothers in my mothers' group just thought I wasn't coping (which to a degree I wasn't) but when their babies cried it was for thirty minutes; Noah cried from morning to night. If he slept in my arms for an hour it was great. I did everything with him in my arms, and was afraid to put him down to go to the toilet. He wouldn't play by himself for more than ten minutes and was so out of whack we didn't know when to bath him, or put him down for the night.*

*Another GP suggested Zantac® as a last-ditch effort after I told her how depressed I was. There was such a marked difference in Noah I couldn't believe it. Sleeps still weren't great but if he was happy in between it was more bearable. We increased Zantac slowly and Noah began sleeping better. We were following a routine and he no longer woke crying.*

*Several weeks ago, we thought he was doing well as he wasn't throwing up much and our paediatrician gave us permission to wean him off medication. Within three days, Noah was crying, arching his back, screaming and sometimes refusing to feed; it was a nightmare and I didn't know what to do. It wasn't until I talked to [another reflux mother] that I realised it was reflux. In hindsight he'd been fussier before we stopped Zantac, but he hadn't done that before and I didn't realise. It took several days on medication to get him settled again . . .*

*We're by no means at the end of our journey, but at least now we have help and support and we know what the problem is. I look back to the twelve hours a day of screaming and nursing him to sleep and look now to the laughing baby and know the journey has been worth it.*

*Kylie*

## Samuel, Millie, Patrick and Jorja

*Samuel projectiled his first 'milk' breastfeed onto the wall. I didn't know what was happening but soon got used to the constant vomiting. He had several apnoeas in the first week, and began screaming. As a first-time mother, I had no idea what had hit me. Sam thankfully slept most nights from sheer exhaustion but I struggled with the idea of routine; going out was difficult and I had extra cleaning as well.*

*We tried positioning/rocking, diet (off dairy but not soy), chiropractors, GPs, paediatricians and medications. I also joined a reflux support group. Sam improved dramatically at around twelve months; however, he still vomits and gags easily, gets carsick and dislikes milk products and raw vegetables/salads (tickling feeling in throat).*

**Millie** *slept on her first day and was a screamer from her second! She had a severe skin rash/eczema, and was diagnosed with colic (she didn't vomit). She didn't sleep well, night or day, and woke or cried at the slightest noise. She was bottle fed from six months – her crying worsened, and she began vomiting. At eight months, Amelia developed a constant cough and was finally diagnosed with asthma.*

*In hindsight, I think Amelia had silent reflux and milk aspiration. Her eczema is still a problem, and she has behaviour problems which have improved dramatically with a diet low in salicylate and amine (food chemicals), no colours/flavours (discovered only recently). Her asthma has improved, but she's allergic to bee stings and several moulds.*

**Patrick** *was the perfect baby and so I experienced a 'normal' baby; very placid, affectionate and an absolute darling. No reflux, colic or constant crying.*

**Jorja** *was born with apnoeas and blue spells and I knew from day one what I was seeing. She cried a lot, had eczema and skin* *rashes like Millie, and vomited once my milk came in. She was diagnosed with reflux at three weeks and put on watch for failure to thrive. She reacted to Losec, so Zantac was prescribed.*

*Some mums suggested I consider going off some foods. My doctor laughed at this, but I was sure I was onto something. With the help of a dietitian, I found she's intolerant to dairy, soy and eggs. Within two weeks on the new diet, her face cleared up, and she no longer vomited. After a month she was off all medication. I test her monthly on her intolerance foods and she still reacts with vomiting or skin reactions. I breastfed her for two and a half years on a restricted diet, and I use a milk replacement for all milk foods and drinks.*

*We've come a long way on our reflux journey. We now know we're an 'atopic' family – hayfever, allergies, asthma and reflux are all symptoms, and that Sam was probably intolerant to milk and soy. I hope our story will encourage others to find medical professionals who listen, and to be confident you are doing the best thing you can for your child at that time with the resources you have available to you.*

*Trudi*

# GLOSSARY

**Allergenic:** substance that causes an allergic reaction

**Anaemia:** not having enough red blood cells and/or haemoglobin (which carry oxygen) in the blood; this can cause symptoms such as tiredness, fatigue and breathlessness

**Anaesthetic:** a drug that causes a temporary loss of feeling or the sensation of pain

>   **General anaesthetic:** a drug that produces loss of consciousness and sensation

**Antacid:** a substance that neutralises acid, especially of the stomach

**Antihistamine:** a drug that blocks the effect of histamine; used for allergy

**Apnoea:** a temporary absence of breathing

>   **Obstructive sleep apnoea:** apnoea that occurs during sleep because of an airway obstruction

**Aspiration:** the act of inhaling foreign matter (e.g. stomach contents) into the lungs

**Asthma:** a chronic lung disorder that causes the air passages to narrow at times, causing symptoms such as wheezing, coughing and/or difficulty breathing

**Barium:** a white liquid that shows up on x-rays

**Barium swallow:** a series of x-rays taken of the upper digestive tract (oesophagus, stomach and small intestine) after a Barium solution is swallowed/ingested

**Barrett's oesophagus:** the presence of changes in cells in the lining of the oesophagus as the body tries to protect itself from chronic reflux; these cells are abnormal and in the long term the risk of developing cancer in the oesophagus may be increased

**Bile:** a greenish fluid that helps in the digestion of fats

**Biopsy:** removal of a small tissue sample from the body for examination under a microscope

**Chronic:** long lasting or recurrent

**Coeliac disease:** a medical condition where there is an intolerance/immune reaction to gluten (a protein in wheat, rye, barley, oats)

**Colic:** a condition of young infants where there are long periods of unexplained crying and irritability; it generally disappears by three months of age

**'Comfort feeder':** a child who wants to feed frequently (as a result of reflux)

**Conservative treatment:** simplest, least invasive treatment (i.e. without medication or surgery)

**Cyanosis:** a bluish skin colour due to a lack of oxygen in the blood

**Developmental milestones:** skills (e.g. physical such as sitting, walking, talking) learnt by most children as they grow and develop

**Digestion:** the process where food is broken down into substances that the body can use

**Digestive tract:** the organs of digestion and elimination, including the mouth, oesophagus, stomach and intestine

**'Dream feed':** a feed given to an infant while they are asleep or drowsy; sometimes done in circumstances when an infant refuses to feed while they are awake

**Duodenum:** the first part of the small intestine, connected to the stomach

**Eczema:** a condition of the skin that can cause itching, scaling and skin thickening

**Endoscope:** a long, flexible, fibre-optic instrument with a light

**Endoscopy:** viewing of a body cavity (e.g. oesophagus) by use of an endoscope

**ENT (ear, nose and throat specialist):** *see Otolaryngologist*

**Enteric coating:** a protective coating on a medication that stops it being broken down as it passes through the stomach, but allows it to break down readily in the intestine; the coating can be around an entire tablet, or around tiny granules in a capsule

**Eustachian tube:** a narrow tube that connects the middle ear to the throat, and helps equalise ear pressure

**Extra-oesophageal reflux:** reflux of gastric juice and acid from the stomach upwards into the oesophagus and then into the mouth, throat or airways

**Failure to thrive (FTT):** faltering growth; a condition where an infant or child's weight or rate of weight gain is significantly below what is expected for their age

**Food allergy:** an immune system response triggered by a specific food; the body identifies the food as being harmful, and creates antibodies to protect itself

**Food intolerance:** the body reacts unpleasantly to a specific food or food additive, but it differs to an allergy as it doesn't involve the immune system

**Fundoplication:** a surgical procedure where the surgeon wraps the top part of the stomach (fundus) around the lower part of the oesophagus as a barrier to reflux

**Gastric:** relating to the stomach

**Gastric emptying:** the action of the stomach emptying its contents into the small intestine; delayed gastric emptying (DGE) is where the stomach empties slower than normal

**Gastric emptying study:** a procedure that uses a small amount of radioactive material to determine the rate food and/or fluids empty from the stomach

**Gastro-oesophageal reflux (GOR):** a condition where the stomach contents flow upwards into the oesophagus (with or without vomiting)

**Gastro-oesophageal reflux disease (GORD):** a disease where gastro-oesophageal reflux causes complications such as oesophagitis, failure to thrive, breathing difficulties or pain

**Gor:** (*see gastro-oesophageal reflux*)

**Gord:** (*see gastro-oesophageal reflux disease*)

**Heartburn:** a painful, burning feeling in the chest; often associated with GOR

**Hiatus hernia:** an opening in the diaphragm (muscle wall between the chest and the abdomen) that allows a portion of the stomach to move into the chest cavity

**Histamine:** a chemical released by the immune system in response to an allergy

**H2 receptor antagonist (H2RA):** acid suppressant medication used in the treatment of reflux

**Hypoallergenic:** substance less likely to cause an allergic reaction

**Indigestion:** a general term that describes stomach discomfort (e.g. bloating, feeling of fullness, nausea, heartburn)

**Infant:** a young child under twelve months of age; a baby

**Infant formula:** an artificial substitute for breastmilk

    **Partially hydrolysed (HA) formula:** an infant formula made of proteins that are partly broken down into smaller molecules

    **Extensively hydrolysed (EHF) formula:** an infant formula made of proteins that are more completely broken down (e.g. Alfaré)

    **Elemental (or amino acid) formula:** a formula made of proteins that are broken down into their most basic level (e.g. EleCare, Neocate)

**Inflammation:** a tissue reaction caused by irritation or injury, which can cause pain, heat, redness, swelling and loss of function in the area

**Laryngo-pharyngeal reflux (LPR):** a condition where the stomach contents flow upwards into the oesophagus and beyond into the mouth and throat

**Lower oesophageal sphincter:** (*see Sphincter*)

**Manometry:** measurement of pressure using specific equipment

**Milk scan:** a medical procedure that tracks radioisotopes given to a child via their breastmilk, formula or food; used to demonstrate evidence of GOR, aspiration and stomach-emptying

**Motility:** refers to the ability of the body to push food through the digestive tract

**Nasogastric (n/g) tube:** a flexible tube placed via the nose and into the stomach; used to empty the stomach, or to pass formula, water and/or medication into it

**Nausea:** refers to the unpleasant sensation of wanting to be sick (vomit).

**Neurological:** relating to the nerves or the nervous system

**Obstructive sleep apnoea:** (*see Apnoea*)

**Oesophagitis:** inflammation of the lining of the oesophagus

**Oesophagus:** the long, hollow, muscular tube that connects the mouth to the stomach; food and fluids travel through the oesophagus to get from the mouth to the stomach

**Oral aversion:** reluctance or refusal to feed or eat

**Otolaryngologist (ENT specialist):** a doctor who specialises in the treatment of diseases of the ears, nose and throat

**Paediatrician:** a doctor who specialises in the treatment of children and infants

**Paediatric gastroenterologist:** a doctor who specialises in treating disorders of the digestive system in infants and children

**Pathological reflux:** reflux that causes injury or disease (*see gastro-oesophageal reflux disease*)

**PEG (percutaneous endoscopic gastrostomy) tube:** a feeding tube inserted directly into the stomach through the abdominal wall; it allows liquid feeds to be put directly into the stomach (percutaneous – through the skin; gastrostomy – surgical opening into the stomach)

**Pepsin:** a stomach enzyme that helps break down protein in the process of digestion

**Peristalsis:** waves of involuntary muscle contractions that assist the passage of food through the digestive system

**pH level:** a measure of acidity or alkalinity of a substance; pH seven is neutral, above seven is alkaline, below seven is acidic

**pH probe:** a medical procedure (often over 24 hours) that measures how often, and for how long, stomach acid flows into the oesophagus

**Physiological reflux:** normal reflux process

**Pneumonia:** inflammation or infection of the lung

**Posset:** to spill back or regurgitate small amounts of milk (without effort)

**Projectile vomiting:** vomiting that forcefully expels stomach contents over some distance

**Prokinetic drugs:** drugs that stimulate movement of the digestive tract

**Prone:** lying face down (on the stomach)

**Proton pump inhibitor (PPI):** acid suppressant medication used in the treatment of reflux; more effective than H2 antagonist medications

**Pyloric sphincter:** (*see Sphincter*)

**Pyloric stenosis:** an obstruction or narrowing at the lower end of the stomach (pylorus); it can cause frequent, forceful vomiting in infants

**Reflux:** a backward flow (*see gastro-oesophageal reflux*)

**Regurgitation:** a backward flow (of food); to bring food up from the stomach without effort

**Respiratory:** relating to breathing

**Sandifer's syndrome:** abnormal head and neck posturing – thought to be in response to pain or the body's way of protecting the airway from reflux

**SIDS:** (*see Sudden Infant Death Syndrome*)

**Signs:** indications of a disease or disorder that can be seen

**Silent reflux:** gastro-oesophageal reflux without any obvious signs (such as vomiting)

**Sphincter:** a ring of muscle that surrounds a natural opening; it opens to allow emptying and closes to prevent backward flow

> **Lower oesophageal sphincter:** sphincter between the oesophagus and stomach

> **Pyloric sphincter:** sphincter located where the stomach and small intestine join

**Stomach:** muscular organ of the digestive tract, found between the oesophagus and small intestine

**Stomach acid:** acid produced in the stomach that aids in the digestion of food

**Stricture:** abnormal narrowing of a passageway, sometimes due to scar tissue

**Stridor:** a harsh sound heard on breathing in (caused by air passing through a narrowed passage)

**Sudden Infant Death Syndrome (SIDS):** a condition where infants die suddenly, for no identifiable reason

**Sudden Unexpected Death in Infancy (SUDI):** sudden and unexpected death of an infant; includes SIDS, fatal sleep accidents and deaths due to illness

**Supine:** lying face up (on the back)

**Surgeon:** a doctor who specialises in surgery

**Symptoms:** indications of a disease or disorder noticed by the patient

**Ulcer:** a break or sore (in the lining of the digestive tract)

**Ulceration:** the formation of an ulcer

**Upper GI series:** (*see Barium swallow*)

**Vomiting:** the forceful expulsion of contents of the stomach through the mouth

**Wheezing:** breathing with a high-pitched whistling sound (often caused when air passes through a narrowed passage)

# SOURCES

Information from Reflux Infants Support Association Inc was used as a basis for this book. Additional information and ideas were collected from the articles and websites listed below.

***

American Academy of Family Physicians 2008, 'Constipation in children', Familydoctor.org, viewed 29 March 2009 <http://family doctor.org/online/famdocen/home/children/parents/common/stomach/222.html>

ANTA 2009, 'Chiropractic', Australian Natural Therapists Association, viewed 15 May 2009 <www.australiannaturaltherapistsassociation.com.au/therapies/chiropractic.php>

Armstrong, KL, et al 1998, 'Sleep deprivation or postnatal depression in later infancy: Separating the chicken from the egg', *Journal of Paediatrics and Child Health*, vol. 34:3, pp. 260–262, viewed 18 November 2008 <www3.interscience.wiley.com/journal/119131966/abstract>

Australian College of Midwives 2007, 'ACM/BFHI position statement. Infant feeding', Australian College of Midwives, viewed 11 November 2009 <www.midwives.org.au/Portals/8/position statements/DRAFT Position Statement on Infant Feeding.pdf>

Bailey, DJ et al 1987, 'Lack of efficacy of thickened feeding as treatment for gastroesophageal reflux', *Journal of Pediatrics*, vol. 110:2, pp. 187–9, viewed 27 August 2009 <www.ncbi.nlm.nih.gov/pubmed/3806288?dopt=Abstract>

# Sources

Beattie, RM 2001, 'Diagnosis and management of gastro-oesophageal reflux', *Current Paediatrics*, vol. 11:4, pp. 269–275.

Boekel, Susan 2007, 'Independent study module. Gastro-esophageal reflux disease (GERD) and the breastfeeding baby', International Lactation Consultant Association, viewed 16 April 2008 <www.ilca.org/education/originalms/GERD.pdf>

Brisbane Osteopathic Centre, 2009, 'Children's health', Brisbane Osteopathic Centre, viewed 20 June 2009 <www.brisbaneosteopathic.com.au/site/children.htm>

Carolina Paediatric Dysphagia 2002, 'Feeding complications of reflux', Carolina Paediatric Dysphagia, viewed 12 February 2009 <www.feeding.com/images/FAQ%20compl%20of%20reflux.doc>

CDHNF 2007, 'Pediatric gastroesophageal reflux. Clinical practice guideline summary' Children's Digestive Health and Nutrition Foundation, viewed 30 April 2008 <http://gerd.cdhnf.org/User/Docs/PDF/GERD_8_pg_brochure_031604.pdf>

CDHNF 2007, 'Pediatric GERD. For most teenagers with GERD, the first step is lifestyle modification', Children's Digestive Health & Nutrition Foundation, viewed 3 May 2008 <http://gerd.cdhnf.org/cms/en/PatientsAndFamilies/Teen/teensacidreflux.aspx?menu=patientsteen>

CDHNF 2007, 'Pediatric GERD. What's up with my kid's stomach?', Children's Digestive Health and Nutrition Foundation, viewed 2 April 2008 <http://gerd.cdhnf.org/cms/en/PatientsAndFamilies/Kids/Patients_Kids_Landing.aspx?menu=patientskids>

CDHNF 2006, 'Teen's checklist for GER or GERD', Children's Digestive Health & Nutrition Foundation, viewed 30 April 2008 <http://gerd.cdhnf.org/User/Docs/pdf/GERDTeenChecklist.pdf>

CDHNF and NASPGHAN 2004, 'Parent's take home guide to GERD', North American Society for Pediatric Gastroenterology and Nutrition, viewed 21 September 2007 <www.naspghan.org/userassets/Documents/pdf/diseaseInfo/GERD-E.pdf>

Children's Hospitals and Clinics of Minnesota 2005, 'GE reflux (milk scan)', Children's Hospitals and Clinics of Minnesota, viewed 21 July 2008 <www.childrensmn.org/Web/Radiology/042065.asp>

Craig, WR et al 2004, 'Metoclopramide, thickened feedings, and positioning for gastro-oesophageal reflux in children under two years (Review)', *Cochrane Database of Systematic Reviews*, issue 3.

Dental Practice Education Research Unit 2006, 'Erosion: Detecting and managing dental erosion', Australian Research Centre for Population Oral Health (ARCPOH), viewed 11 November 2009 <www.arcpoh.adelaide.edu.au/dperu/special/erosion/Erosion A3.pdf>

Diamant, Nicholas E 2006, 'Pathophysiology of gastroesophageal reflux disease', GI Motility Online, viewed 29 March 2008 <www.nature.com/gimo/contents/pt1/full/gimo21.html>

DISA 2001, 'Dealing with health professionals', DISA, viewed 18 November 2006 <http://home.vicnet.net.au/~disa/ Dealing%20with%20Professionals.html>

Elkins, K n.d., 'Thesis summary: the psychosocial impact of caring for an infant suffering from reflux'.

Gaffney, Kathleen F 2001, 'Infant exposure to environmental tobacco smoke', *Journal of Nursing Scholarship*, vol. 33:4, pp. 343–347, viewed 21 July 2008, <www3.interscience.wiley.com/journal/118999861/abstract>

Gillson, Sharon 2008, 'Meal planning quick tips to prevent heartburn', About.com: Heartburn/GERD, viewed 12 September 2008 <http://heartburn.about.com/od/goodfoodsbadfoods/qt/mealplanningtip.htm>

Gold, Benjamin D 2004, 'Gastroesophageal reflux disease: Could intervention in childhood reduce the risk of later complications?', *The American Journal of Medicine*, vol. 117:5, pp. 23S-29S.

Gremse, David A 2004, 'GERD in the pediatric patient: Management considerations', Medscape Pediatrics, viewed 20 October 2009 <www.medscape.com/viewarticle/472765_print>

## Sources

Heacock, Helen J et al 1992, 'Influence of breast versus formula milk on physiological gastroesophageal reflux in healthy, newborn infants', *Journal of Pediatric Gastroenterology and Nutrition*, vol. 14:1, pp. 41–6.

HealthyMedicine.com.au 2009, 'Naturopathy', Healthy Medicine, viewed 16 October 2009 <http://healthymedicine.net.au/naturopathy/naturopathy.htm>

Henry, Shawna 2004, 'Discerning differences: Gastroesophageal reflux and gastroesophageal reflux disease in infants', *Advances in Neonatal Care*, vol. 4:4, pp. 235-247.

Holloway, Richard H & Orenstein, Susan R 1991, 'Gastro-oesophageal reflux disease in adults and children', *Baillière's Clinical Gastroenterology*, vol. 5:2, pp. 337–370.

Homeopathy Clinic 2008, 'Frequently asked questions', Homeopathy Works, viewed 19 June 2009 <www.homeopathyworks.com.au/faq.html>

Infant Massage Information Service 2009, 'About – benefits', IMIS – Infant Massage Information Service, viewed 20 June 2009 <www.infantmassage-imis.com.au/info.asp?page_id=7>

Kawahara, H, Dent, J, & Davidson, G 1997, 'Mechanisms responsible for gastroesophageal reflux in children', *Gastroenterology*, vol. 113:2, pp. 399–408, viewed 22 October 2009 <www.gastrojournal.org/article/S0016-5085(97)00361-2/abstract>

Kemp, Andrew S et al 2008, 'Guidelines for the use of infant formulas to treat cows milk protein allergy: An Australian consensus panel opinion', *Medical Journal of Australia*, vol. 188, pp. 109–112, viewed 18 November 2008 <www.mcri.edu.au/Downloads/Media/2008/02/01/Article7.pdf>

Kiwanis Club of Ottawa 2008, 'About shaken baby syndrome', Never Shake a Baby, viewed 27 May 2008 <www.nevershakeababy.org/about>

Krishnan, Usha et al 2002, 'Assay of tracheal pepsin as a marker of reflux aspiration', *Journal of Pediatric Gastroenterology and*

*Nutrition*, vol. 35:3, pp. 303-308, viewed 24 July 2008 <http://pdfs.journals.lww.com/jpgn/2002/09000/Assay_of_Tracheal_Pepsin_as_a_Marker_of_Reflux.12.pdf>

Lawlor-Smith, Carolyn 2005, 'Unsettled breastfed babies', Southern Division of General Practice, viewed 20 May 2008 <www.sdgp.com.au/client_images/18177.pdf>

Lifschitz, Carlos 2009, 'Patient information: Gastroesophageal reflux disease in children and adolescents', UpToDate.for patients, viewed 16 November 2009 <www.uptodate.com/patients/content/topic.do?topicKey=~ousooi.n/Gl.Qgs>

Linnett, V et al 2002, 'Oral health of children with gastro-esophageal reflux disease: A controlled study', *Australian Dental Journal*, vol. 47:2, pp. 156-162, viewed 25 July 2008 <www.ada.org.au/App_CmsLib/Media/Lib/0610/M28722_v1_632973619167160000.pdf>

Mathisen, B et al 1999, 'Feeding problems in infants with gastro-oesophageal reflux disease: A controlled study', *Journal of Paediatrics and Child Health*, vol. 35:2, pp. 163–9

Mathisen, B and Shepherd, R 1995, 'Communication at mealtimes in infants with gastro-oesophageal reflux', Australian Early Intervention Association (NSW Chapter) Conference

McLoughlin, Heidi 2008, 'How to use infant massage to relieve reflux', How to Do Things.com, viewed 20 June 2009 <www.howtodothings.com/family-relationships/how-to-use-infant-massage-to-relieve-reflux>

Medicines Talk 2008, 'Keeping a lid on medicine costs', *Medicines Talk*, no. 25, pp. 1–3.

Moazzez, R, Bartlett, D, & Anggiansah, A 2005, 'The effect of chewing sugar-free gum on gastro-esophageal reflux', *Journal of Dental Research*, vol. 84:11, pp. 1062–1065, viewed 21 July 2008 <http://jdr.sagepub.com/cgi/content/full/84/11/1062>

Mohammed, Asim A et al 2005, 'Association of food and drinks with gastroesophageal reflux symptoms in adolescents', *Journal of*

*Pediatric Gastroenterology and Nutrition*, vol. 41:4, p. 504, viewed July 25 2008 <http://journals.lww.com/jpgn/Fulltext/2005/10000/Association_Of_Food_And_Drinks_With.61.aspx>

myDr 2002, 'Naturopathy', myDr, viewed 15 May 2009 <www.mydr.com.au/complementary-medicine/naturopathy>

NDDIC 2006, 'Gastroesophageal reflux in children and adolescents', National Digestive Diseases Information Clearinghouse, viewed 28 March 2008 <http://digestive.niddk.nih.gov/ddiseases/pubs/gerinchildren/index.htm>

NDDIC 2006, 'Gastroesophageal reflux in infants', National Digestive Diseases Information Clearinghouse, viewed 28 March 2008 <http://digestive.niddk.nih.gov/ddiseases/pubs/gerdinfant/index.htm>

NDDIC 2007, 'Heartburn, gastroesophageal reflux (GER) and gastroesophageal reflux disease (GERD)', National Digestive Diseases Information Clearinghouse, viewed 2 Feb 2008 <http://digestive.niddk.nih.gov/ddiseases/pubs/gerd/>

Nelson, Suzanne P et al 1998, 'One-year follow-up of symptoms of gastroesophageal reflux during infancy', *Pediatrics*, vol. 102:6, p. e67, viewed 18 November 2008 <http://pediatrics.aappublications.org/cgi/content/full/102/6/e67>

NHMRC, 2003, 'Dietary guidelines for children and adolescents in Australia', National Health & Medical Research Council, viewed 17 September 2009 <www.nhmrc.gov.au/_files_nhmrc/file/publications/synopses/n34.doc>

Orenstein, Susan R 1992, 'Gastroesophageal reflux', *Pediatrics in Review*, vol. 13, pp. 174–182, viewed 23 July 2008 <http://pedsinreview.aappublications.org/cgi/content/abstract/13/5/174>

Orenstein, SR 2007, 'Pediatric erosive esophagitis maintenance: Finally, some level 1 evidence!', *American Journal of Gastroenterology*, Vol. 102:6, pp. 1298-300. viewed 9 Nov 2009 <www.mdconsult.com/das/journal/view/0/N/19671749?issn=&source=MI>

Orenstein, Susan R, Izadnia, Fariba, & Khan, Seema 1999, 'Gastroesophageal reflux disease in children', *Gastroenterology Clinics of North America*, vol. 28:4, pp. 947-969, viewed 29 March 2008 <www.sciencedirect.com/science?_ob=ArticleURL&_udi=B75J6-4G7WVC5-D&_user=10&_rdoc=1&_fmt=&_orig=search&_sort=d&view=c&_acct=C000050221&_version=1&_urlVersion=0&_userid=10&md5=94539732baba2628c8f0f6cca9dcb656>

Orenstein, SR & McGowan, JD 2008, 'Efficacy of conservative therapy as taught in the primary care setting for symptoms suggesting infant gastroesophageal reflux', *Journal of Pediatrics*, vol. 152:3, pp. 310–314, viewed 21 July 2008 <www.ncbi.nlm.nih.gov/pubmed/18280832>

Orenstein, SR et al 2006, 'Natural history of infant reflux esophagitis: Symptoms and morphometric histology during one year without pharmacotherapy'. *American Journal of Gastroenterology*, vol. 101:3, pp. 628-40, viewed 23 July 2008 <www.ncbi.nlm.nih.gov/pubmed/16542296>

Persing, John et al 2003, 'Prevention and management of positional skull deformities in infants', *Pediatrics*, vol. 112:1, pp. 199–202, viewed 21 July 2008 <http://pediatrics.aappublications.org/cgi/content/full/112/1/199>

Queensland Health & SIDS and Kids 2008, 'Tummy playtime', Queensland Health, viewed 10 April 2009 <www.health.qld.gov.au/ph/documents/childhealth/TummyPlay_Brochure.pdf>

Queensland Health 2008, 'Safe infant care to reduce the risk of sudden unexpected deaths in infancy: Policy statement and guidelines', Queensland Health, viewed 7 October 2009 <www.health.qld.gov.au/ph/documents/childhealth/29567.pdf>

Richter, Joel 1999, 'Do we know the cause of reflux disease?', *European Journal of Gastroenterology and Hepatology*, vol. 11:1, pp. S3–9, viewed 22 October 2009 <http://journals.lww.com/eurojgh/pages/articleviewer.aspx?year=1999&issue=06001&article=00002&type=abstract>

Rodríguez, Parilla et al 2002, 'Knowledge about breastfeeding in mothers of infants with gastroesophageal reflux', *Puerto Rico Health Sciences Journal*, vol. 21:1, pp. 25–9.

Rosen, Frederick S and Friedman, Normal R 2000, 'Pediatric gastroesophageal reflux', Dept. of Otolaryngology, University of Texas Medical Branch, viewed 20 March 2008 <www.utmb.edu/otoref/Grnds/Pedi-GERD-0010/Pedi-gerd-001025.htm>

Salvatore, Silvia & Vandenplas, Yvan 2002, 'Gastroesophageal reflux and cow milk allergy: Is there a link?', *Pediatrics*, vol. 110:5, pp. 972–984, viewed 15 August 2006 <http://pediatrics.aap publications.org/cgi/content/full/110/5/972>

Schwartz, Richard H & Bahadori, Robert A 2006, 'The adenoid in children: Out of sight, out of mind?', Pediatric Supersite, viewed 27 August 2009 <www.pediatricsupersite.com/view.aspx?rid= 36199>

Schwarz, Steven M & Hebra, Andre 2009, 'Gastroesophageal reflux', eMedicine, viewed 26 August 2009 <http://emedicine. medscape.com/article/930029-print>

Shabib, Souheil M, 1995, 'Passive smoking is a risk factor for esophagitis in children', *Journal of Pediatrics*, vol. 127:3, pp. 435–437, viewed 2 November 2009 <www.jpeds.com/article/S0022-3476(95)70078-1/abstract>

Shepherd, RW et al 1987, 'Gastroesophageal reflux in children'. *Clinical Pediatrics*, vol. 26:2, pp. 55–60, viewed 25 July 2008 <http://cpj.sagepub.com/cgi/content/abstract/26/2/55>

Sherman, Philip M et al 2004, 'Sharing solutions in pediatric gastroenterology: Building algorithms for gastro-esophageal reflux disease', Medscape CME, viewed 2 April 2008 <http://cme.medscape.com/viewarticle/494079_print>

SIDS and Kids 2008, 'Information statement: Wrapping babies', SIDS and Kids, viewed 9 May 2009 <www.sidsandkids.org/documents/WrappingBabiesInfostatementOctober2008.pdf>

SIDS and Kids 2009, 'Sudden unexpected death in infancy (SUDI):

Frequently asked questions', SIDS and Kids, viewed 23 October 2009 <www.sidsandkids.org/documents/2009_03FAQMarch 2009.pdf>

SIDS and Kids 2007 'Information statement. Sleeping with a baby', SIDS and Kids, viewed 21 July 2008 <www.sidsandkids.org/ documents/SleepingwithababyInformationStatement.pdf>

Skopnik, Heino et al 1996, 'Gastroesophageal reflux in infants: Evaluation of a new intraluminal impedance technique', *Journal of Pediatric Gastroenterology & Nutrition*, vol. 23:5, pp. 591-598, viewed 18 November 2008 <www.jpgn.org/pt/re/jpgn/full-text.00005176-199612000-00014.htm;jsessionid=LJscryFJXRpL Hbbs4Jy48H9TrKGfq5t2yM5BWnqQxQbJ80llpFV4!52380700 9!181195628!8091!-1>

Sondheimer, Judith M 2005, 'Gastroesophageal reflux', Children's Hospital and Regional Medical Center, viewed 25 March 2008 <www.pediatricweb.com/seattle/article.asp?ArticleID=811& ArticleType=9>

Stanciu, C & Bennett, John R 1972, 'Smoking and gastro-oesophageal reflux', *British Medical Journal*, vol. 3, pp. 793–795, viewed 21 July 2008 <http://ukpmc.ac.uk/articlerender.cgi? artid=885809>

Strudwick, Sue 2003, 'Gastro-oesophageal reflux and feeding: The speech and language therapist's perspective', *International Journal of Pediatric Otorhinolaryngology*, vol. 67S1, pp. S101–S102.

Vandenplas, Yvan et al 1998, 'Nutritional management of regurgitation in infants', *Journal of the American College of Nutrition*, vol. 17:4, pp. 308–316, viewed 20 March 2008 <www.jacn.org/cgi/ content/full/17/4/308>

Vandenplas, Yvan et al 2009, 'Pediatric gastroesophageal reflux clinical practice guidelines: Joint recommendations of NASPGHAN and ESPGHAN', *Journal of Pediatric Gastroenterology and Nutrition*, vol. 49:4, pp. 498–547, viewed 31 October 2009

<http://journals.lww.com/jpgn/Fulltext/2009/10000/Pediatric_Gastroesophageal_Reflux_Clinical.22.aspx>

von Schönfeld, JV et al 1997, 'Oesophageal acid and salivary secretion: Is chewing gum a treatment option for gastro-oesophageal reflux?', *Digestion*, vol. 58:2, pp. 111–114, viewed 21 July 2008 <http://content.karger.com/ProdukteDB/produkte.asp?Doi=201432>

West, Nicola X 2007, 'The dentine hypersensitivity patient – a total management package', *International Dental Journal*, vol. 57, pp. 411-419.

Winston, Anthony P, Hardwick, Elizabeth, & Jaberi, Neema 2005, 'Neuropsychiatric effects of caffeine', *Advances in Psychiatric Treatment*, vol. 11, pp. 432–439, viewed 4 May 2008 <http://apt.rcpsych.org/cgi/content/full/11/6/432>

Winter, Harland S 2009, 'Patient information: Gastroesophageal reflux in infants', UpToDate. for patients, viewed 16 November 2009 <www.uptodate.com/patients/content/topic.do?topicKey=~q7OOqbN6FY8NphO>

Wynyard Chiropractic 2009, 'Cry baby', Wynyard Chiropractic, viewed 22 August 2009 <www.wynyardchiro.com.au/Articles/Paediatriccare/Crybaby/tabid/160/Default.aspx>

# Notes on Contributors
# and Reviewers

The following health professionals made valuable contributions to this book by reviewing articles and/or writing them. Special thanks to Joan Breakey, Dr Julie Cichero and Dr Jeanine Young for allowing their work to be included in the book and for their time.

**Professor Terry Bolin**, MD(NSW) BS(Syd) FRACP FRCP(Lond) FRCP(Edin) DCH(Lond), Gastroenterologist, Conjoint Associate Professor of Medicine, University of New South Wales, Consultant Emeritus to the Gastrointestinal Unit, Prince of Wales Hospital, Sydney, President, Gut Foundation – *reviewed Chapter 1, Chapter 2, 'Bowel Disturbances', Glossary*

**Joan Breakey**, M App Sc, BSc, Cert Diet, DNFS, TTTC Specialist Dietitian Allergy & Food Sensitivity – *wrote 'Introducing Solids to a Reflux Infant', 'Some Important Ideas to Help Prevent Fussy Eaters', 'Is Your Reflux Infant (or Older Child) Food Sensitive?'; reviewed 'General Management Strategies for Giving Solids', 'Thickened Feeds/Food Thickeners', 'Introduction to Food Sensitivities'*

**Fiona Carter**, B.App.Sci.(Biol/Biotech) hons., Dip.Clin.Nut. – *reviewed 'Biomedical Intervention and Nutrition'*

**Professor Anthony G Catto-Smith**, MB BS, MD, FRACP, MRCP, DCH, AGAF, Director of Gastroenterology and Clinical

Nutrition, Royal Children's Hospital, Melbourne – *reviewed 'What Causes Reflux and its Complications?', 'What does Reflux look like?', 'Complications of Reflux', 'Growing out of Reflux', 'Common Myths about Reflux in Children', 'Reflux is not Always to Blame', 'When to Especially Seek Medical Advice', 'Multichannel Intraluminal Impedance (MII)/pH Monitoring', 'Tracheal Pepsin Assay', 'ALTE'*

**Felicity Chapman**, B.Soc.W. (Hons), Assoc.Dip.C.Counselling – *wrote 'Living with Reflux: Ethan and Tyler'; reviewed Chapter 14*

**Dr Julie Cichero**, BA, BSpThy (Hons) PhD, Senior Research Fellow and Honorary Research Consultant with the University of Queensland (previously of Pero Clinic, and No Fuss Feeding and Swallowing Centre) – *wrote 'Concerns Regarding Infant Feeding Patterns', 'GOR and Feeding Development', 'Everyday Feeding-Related Activities for Children', 'Speech Pathology Questions and Answers'; reviewed 'Modified Barium Swallow', 'Feeding Difficulties in Breast and Bottle Fed Infants', 'Comfort Feeding', 'Feeding Issues in Children on Solids', 'Other Developmental Issues'*

**Robyn Crapp**, RN, Nurse Unit Manager, Medical Imaging Department, The Children's Hospital at Westmead – *reviewed 'Barium Swallow'*

**Mary da Silva**, RN, RM, Ba. Nursing, Nurse Unit Manager, Gastroenterology Unit, Royal Children's Hospital, Brisbane – *reviewed 'Discussing Issues with your Doctor', 'Fasting for Investigations', 'Upper Endoscopy', 'pH probe', 'Oesophageal Manometry', 'General Home Management Tips', Chapter 14, Chapter 15*

**Professor Elizabeth Elliott**, MD MPhil FRACP FRCPCH FRCP, Professor of Paediatrics and Child Health, University of Sydney, Consultant Paediatrician, The Children's Hospital at Westmead, Head, Centre for Evidence Based Paediatrics, Gastroenterology and Nutrition – *reviewed 'Eosinophilic Oesophagitis'*

**Dr Hashem B. El-Serag**, MD, MPH, Professor of Medicine, Chief, Gastroenterology and Hepatology Section, Dept. of Medicine, Chief, Clinical Epidemiology and Outcomes, Health Services Research, Michael E DeBakey VA Medical Center & Baylor College of Medicine, Texas – *reviewed 'Asthma', 'Bowel Disturbances'*

**Associate Professor Roger Hall OAM**, MDSC FRACDS FICD, Paediatric Dental Surgeon, Principal Fellow (Hon.) Department Of Pharmacology, University Of Melbourne; Emeritus Dental Surgeon, Royal Children's Hospital, Melbourne – *reviewed 'Teeth Issues'*

**Leonie Helder**, Bowen Therapist, member BTAWA/BTFA – *reviewed 'Bowen Therapy'*

**Associate Professor Andrew Holland**, BSc (Hons) MB BS PhD (Syd) Grad Cert Ed Studies (Higher Ed) FRCS (Eng) FRACS (Paed), Paediatric Surgeon, Director, Burns Research Institute, Department of Academic Surgery, The Children's Hospital at Westmead, University of Sydney – *reviewed Chapter 11, Chapter 12*

**Professor Robert Howman-Giles**, MB BS MD FRACP DDU, Head, Department of Nuclear Medicine, The Children's Hospital at Westmead – *reviewed 'Milk Scan'*

**Kay Hynes**, BPharm, DipClinPharm, Senior Pharmacist, Drug Information & Clinical Trials, Pharmacy Department, Royal Children's Hospital, Melbourne – *reviewed Chapter 9*

**Julie Maddox**, RN, RM, CFHN, Masters in Nursing Clinical Leadership, Clinical Nurse Consultant, Child and Family Health – *reviewed 'Common Characteristics of Reflux', 'Breast and Formula Feeding', 'Strategies for Feeding Difficulties', 'Strategies for Comfort Feeding', 'General Management Strategies for Giving Solids'*

**Dr Sarah Manns**, PhD, MSc, LLb (Hons), Research Fellow, Centre for Clinical and Health Services Research, School of Health and Social Care, University of the West of England – *reviewed Chapter 3, Chapter 4, Chapter 5, Chapter 11, Chapter 15*

**Dr David Manton**, BDSc, MDSc, FRACDS, Senior Lecturer Growth and Development & Paediatric Dentistry, Convenor, Paediatric Dentistry Program, Melbourne Dental School, University of Melbourne – *reviewed 'Teeth Issues'*

**Heidi McLoughlin**, CIMI; AITIM, Infant Massage Trainer, Infant Massage Information Service – *reviewed 'Infant Massage'*

**Christine Plover**, BPharm (Hons), MClinPharm, Pharmacist, Drug Information & Clinical Trials Pharmacy Department, Royal Children's Hospital, Melbourne – *reviewed Chapter 9*

**Trent Sigley**, B.App.Sc. (Clin Sc), B.Ost.Sc., Osteopath, Brisbane Osteopathic Centre – *assisted with writing 'Osteopathy'*

**Kylie Simpson**, BSc. DBM. DRM, Naturopath – *reviewed Chapter 10*

**Dr Shyan Vijayasekaran**, MBBS, FRACS, Otolaryngologist Head and Neck Surgeon, Princess Margaret Hospital for Children, Clinical Associate Professor, University of Western Australia – *reviewed 'ENT (Ear, Nose and Throat) Conditions'*

**Dr Heidi Webster**, MBBS, FRACP, MPH, Community Paediatrician, Royal Children's Hospital & Health Service District – *reviewed 'Asthma', 'Bowel Disturbances', 'ALTE'*

**Professor (Adjunct) Jeanine Young**, FRCNA, PhD BSc (Hons) Adv Diploma Nursing, RGN EM Neonatal Nurse, Nursing Director – Research, Royal Children's Hospital and Health Service, Children's Health Service District, Adjunct Professor, Research Centre for Clinical and Community Practice Innovation, Griffith University, Adjunct Associate Professor, School of Nursing and Midwifery, Queensland University of Technology, Adjunct Associate Professor, University of Queensland, School of Nursing and Midwifery – *wrote 'Positioning for Sleep' and 'Additional*

*Settling Strategies'; reviewed Chapter 3, Chapter 4, Chapter 5, Chapter 11, Chapter 15*